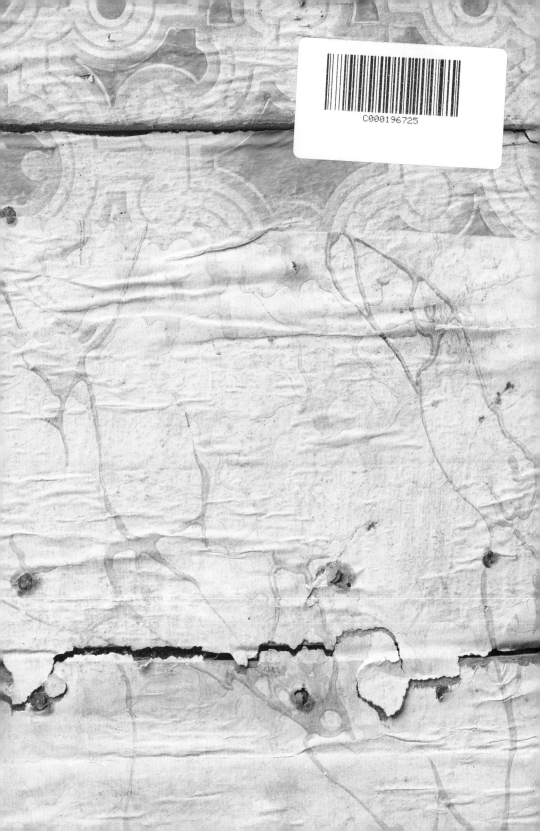

Gentle Spells & Kind Magic

Sam McKechnie

PAVILION

For my mum

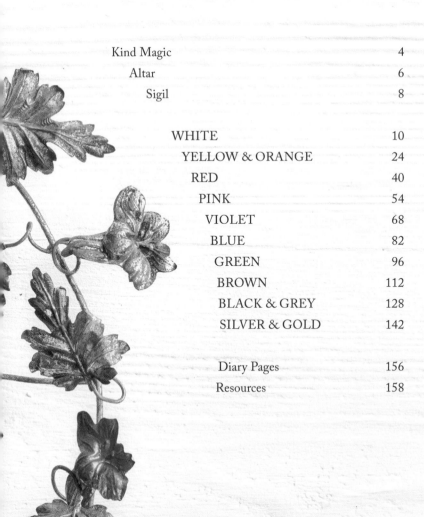

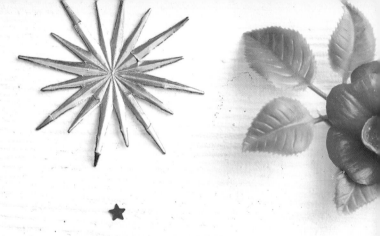

Kind Magic

I have always believed in magic. My mother did too, and her family before her. Magic had a natural place in our everyday life – from casting spells with salt to protect the house, to charming my friend's warts, to keeping lucky charms in our coat pockets. I cannot remember a time I didn't believe.

Magic, for me, can take many forms, whether it be a desire, a wish, or a spell. It can even be a simple act of kindness for friends and family and, importantly, for yourself too – like a lovingly handmade gift or comforting plate of food! So here you'll find a collection of gentle spells and charms, rituals and recipes, poems and crafts.

Magic can even be a gesture: a recognition of emotion in others; a helping hand; a kind word to a stranger. Reaching out to others, even in a simple way – like telling someone that you think they are beautiful or that they have brightened your day with their smile – is a powerful force for good. Be generous in life and be kind, without expectation.

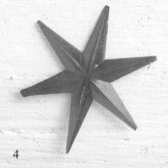

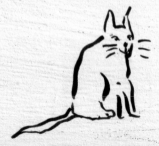

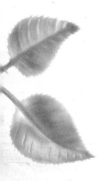

Gentle Spells & Good Intentions

My hope when writing this book was to provide a gentle form of magic with crystal-clear instructions, to allow you to create magic for yourself. The most important element of magic is clarity. Particularly when making your intention. An intention is simply your aim, a crystallization of your desire. Each chapter of this book is based on a colour, which is a wonderful way to curate and organize what you feel and need.

On page 6, I show you how to create an altar. This is a place where you can concentrate and focus while making your intention. You can decorate it with flowers, crystals and gems, and symbols of the element (earth, fire, air, water) associated with a particular colour. But don't worry if an altar isn't for you – you can make magic anywhere.

As with every person, every witch is unique. This book cannot, and indeed will not, tell you what to do. Only you know the spells and intentions that are right for you. Try not to make magic when upset, distressed or ill, as this may muddy your intention. And never make magic that could coerce or influence another. Kindness is at the heart of this magic and it is not intended to be used negatively in any way.

THIS MAGIC IS FOR YOU.

I hope that this book will either start your adventure into magic or validate your magical beliefs to open a whole new world.

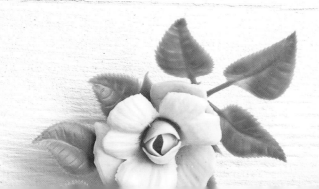

Altar

An altar, or mantle, should be a beautiful place that makes you feel calm and clear. It is an important space for you to breathe and focus on your intentions. I have always made small altars, even as a young child. Collections of flowers, herbs, feathers, rocks, crystals and treasured objects representative of figures in my life, have always been important to me. It feels instinctive and natural to have a special place in my home for these cherished items. These magical spaces can take many forms – they can be fancy or simple, showy or discreet. As long as you have a dedicated, intimate space they can be made anywhere – in any room, outside in the garden, on a table, on a mantelpiece or even on the corner of a shelf.

Traditionally, altars are decorated in keeping with the natural ebb and flow of the seasons. Just as the seasons change, our needs, and therefore our intentions, often change in step with them. We may need strength and comfort through the darker winter months or confidence for a fresh start in spring. I particularly like to harness the power of colour to decorate my altar, and have suggested flowers, crystals, gems and elements in every chapter to help you unlock the magic of colour.

Another traditional decoration for an altar is a pentagram. (A pentagram is a five-pointed star and the five points represent 'Spirit', 'Earth', 'Fire', 'Water' and 'Air'.) A pentagram is a talisman of protection. A pentacle is a pentagram with a protective circle, enclosing the star.

Historically the four elements are also represented. Earth is placed to the north of the altar. You can represent it with a little soil, a crystal or a fossil. Air is placed to the east, represented by a feather, or perhaps some incense. Fire is placed to the south, represented by a candle or match. Water is placed to the west, represented by a bowl of water or a shell.

It's important to remember that this information isn't intended as a to-do list or a strict set of instructions. Your altar or mantle is for you and you alone. Gather the objects that are special to you. You can add photographs of people passed, or of friends and family members who are in your thoughts.

Wherever you decide to make your altar and however you decide to decorate it, make sure you keep the magic alive by dusting it regularly, keeping it uncluttered and relevant to how you are feeling or to the type of magic you want to work. Use fresh water, flowers and herbs, and new candles for each spell. Although, if you are reworking an old spell that's intention is the same, it's fine to use your original candle.

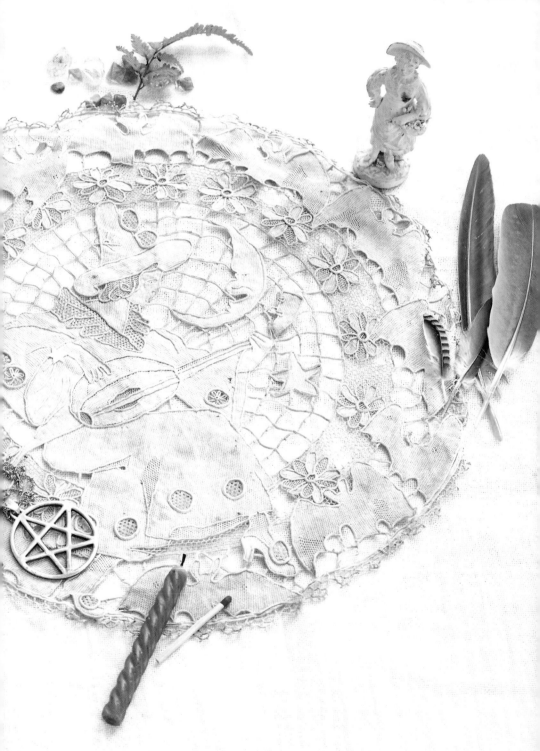

Sigil

A sigil is an intention condensed into a symbol – they are a wonderful form of magic. Whether they are complicated and mysterious or simple and beautiful, they are hugely powerful (formed by your own secret purpose), and can only be deciphered by the person that creates them.

There are several ways to create a sigil, but the following method is straightforward and clear, and requires minimal tools, which I prefer.

When making a sigil, make your intention an immediate, positive affirmation, such as I AM STRONG, rather than I WANT TO BE STRONG or I WISH TO BE STRONG or GIVE ME STRENGTH!

First write down your statement, intention or wish…

I AM STRONG

Next, remove all the vowels and any repeated letters…

~~I~~ **~~A~~M STR~~O~~NG**

Look at the letters you are left with…
M S T R N G

Now use these letters to make a symbol. Play with them. Be creative (you can use ink, paint or pencils to create your symbol) and consider your intention. Do you associate it with a particular colour – red for strength or love, blue for reflection and tranquillity?

You could also decorate your sigil by adding arrows, stars, moons… whatever feels right.

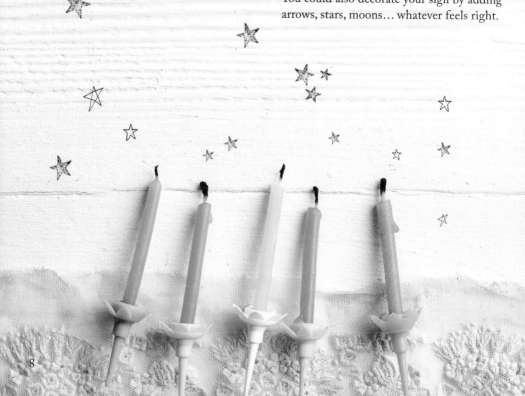

How does your sigil look? Is it strong? Does it lift you? Does it make your heart sing?

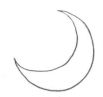

Take a moment to breathe and consider your sigil. Be certain your intention is correct. Once you're happy with your sigil, draw it on a piece of paper and keep it in a safe place or begin a sigil diary – you'll find space to do just that on pages 156–157. Sigils can be used multiple times or until you feel the need for a new one.

There are many ways for these potent symbols to be activated. Choose what feels right for you.

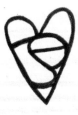

* Draw the sigil on your hand or wrist in a colour that strengthens your intention. As it fades each time you wash your hands, your wish or intention will manifest.

* Etch your sigil onto a coloured candle using a pin. As the candle burns, your wish is free to manifest.

* Draw your sigil on a piece of paper and pop it under a tea light.

* Draw your sigil on a piece of paper and carry it in your pocket, locket or bag.

* Embroider your sigil onto your clothes or handkerchief.

* Draw a sigil on a pebble and leave it on the beach for the sea to wash over.

* Draw your sigil in the condensation on a mirror – as the mirror clears, your intention will manifest.

* Draw your sigil in earth, sand or snow, and ask Mother Earth (the personification of nature) to help your intention or wish manifest.

* Draw your sigil on paper and add it to the tinder of your fire before setting it alight. Alternatively, burn your sigil in a bonfire or flame. When burning your sigil, make sure you've kept a record as the paper will be gone in a flash. Copy it into your notebook or sigil diary alongside the date, so you can see when your intention manifests.

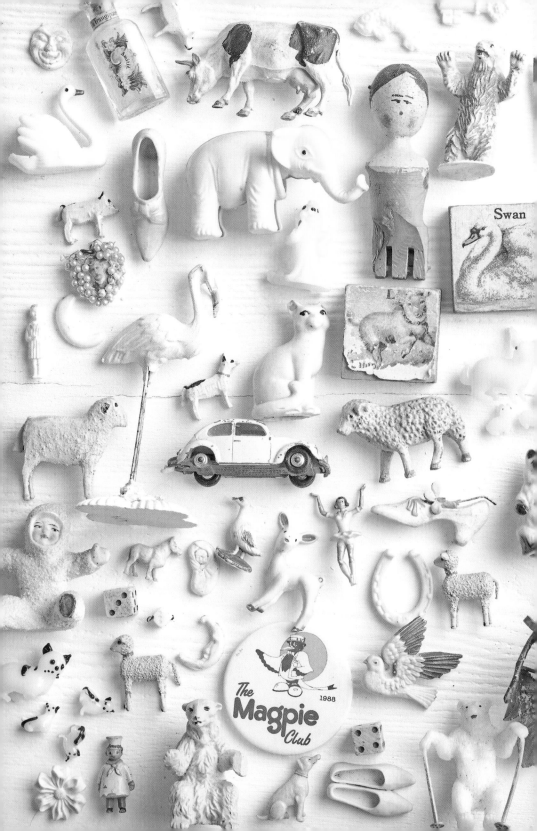

Swan

The Magpie Club 1988

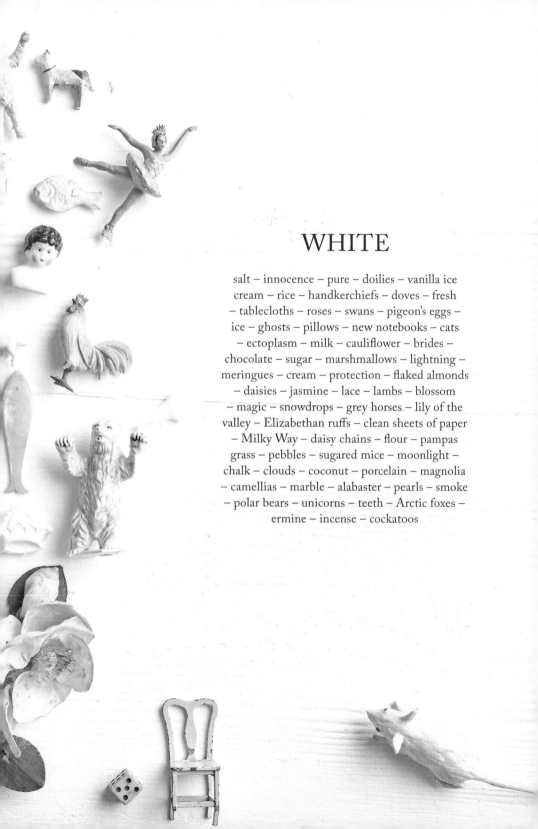

WHITE

salt – innocence – pure – doilies – vanilla ice
cream – rice – handkerchiefs – doves – fresh
– tablecloths – roses – swans – pigeon's eggs –
ice – ghosts – pillows – new notebooks – cats
– ectoplasm – milk – cauliflower – brides –
chocolate – sugar – marshmallows – lightning –
meringues – cream – protection – flaked almonds
– daisies – jasmine – lace – lambs – blossom
– magic – snowdrops – grey horses – lily of the
valley – Elizabethan ruffs – clean sheets of paper
– Milky Way – daisy chains – flour – pampas
grass – pebbles – sugared mice – moonlight –
chalk – clouds – coconut – porcelain – magnolia
– camellias – marble – alabaster – pearls – smoke
– polar bears – unicorns – teeth – Arctic foxes –
ermine – incense – cockatoos

WHITE

White is a colour of simplicity and quiet, and is the best colour to help you focus on intentions and rituals that concern protection or encouragement.

White is also considered to be the colour of innocence. During the Renaissance, white unicorns were revered as a symbol of chastity. These wild, mysterious and elusive creatures were believed to have a horn of such magic and purity that famous hunts were organized to capture these beautiful beasts. (These hunts were immortalized in exquisite woven tapestries.)

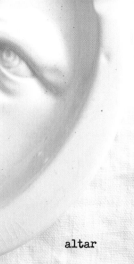

altar

flower: daisies, snowdrops, chrysanthemums
crystals & gems: pearl, rock crystal
element: air

White can also help you to restore a sense of order and efficiency in your life. It can declutter or cleanse a space, encouraging you to let go of negative energy and emotions to leave you feeling 'lighter' and hopeful. The colour can also soothe and calm – imagine the feeling of crisp white bedsheets and clean white night clothes before a restful night's sleep.

It's also a great colour to represent a fresh start or new beginning. Think of a beautiful bride garlanded in pure white blossom. Or remember the excitement of starting a new notebook at the beginning of the school term? Symbolically, white is extremely powerful, giving you both a wonderful free rein and the strength to define your boundaries – draw a line in the sand, run upon that white snow and make your mark on a blank canvas.

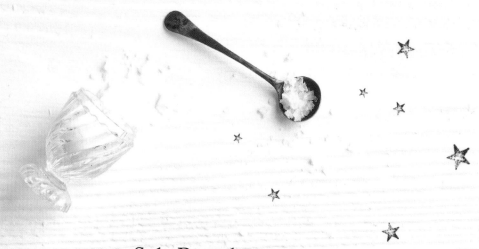

Salt Rituals

Salt is a simple, everyday staple for cooking, yet it's also an essential tool for everyday magic. Salt has always been believed to have magical, protective and purifying qualities, and is thought to absorb negative psychic energies too.

In ancient times, salt was considered a valuable commodity, only the wealthy could afford it and the Romans even paid their soldiers in salt. Salt has long been used to purify spaces and repel negative energy. Across the British Isles and Europe in the 1600s, salt would be sprinkled around butter churns to keep malevolent sprites from souring the milk. Salt was also used in a complex ritual performed over the heads of children said to have been bewitched or captured by fairies.

There are certain speciality salts that you can buy specifically for spells, but I use the same salt for my cooking and my magic – both are daily pleasures. I believe you can use any type of salt for these rituals, but as I am a water lover, sea salt is the one that resonates for me.

Simple Salt Cleanse

Sometimes other people's negativity and toxic energy can be dumped on us. Whether this is intentional or accidental, it can make us feel quite heavy. Of course, we can dump lots of negative thoughts and downright cruelties on ourselves and others too. A salt cleanse will remove negative energy for a short while and bring clarity to your thoughts. It's so simple and can easily become a daily ritual that can help you to feel as light and fresh as washing your face with cold, clear water.

Take a pinch of salt.

Encircle the crown of your head in a clockwise motion.

Let the salt fall away with a flick of your hand.

Let negative energy fall away with the salt and whisper, 'Be gone'.

Allow yourself to be quiet for a moment…

How do you feel?

Are you okay?

Do you have more negative feelings you
need to let go of?

Draw or write down how you are feeling.

Home Sweet Home

A magic circle, often made with salt, is used to protect those
within it. When making magic, to feel clear and truly understand
your intention, it may help to sprinkle a circle of salt around you,
with you in the centre.

To help protect your home from negativity, you can sprinkle salt
across its portals – your doorways, windows and hearths.

Focus on your intention, 'I am protected'.

Sprinkle salt across your front and back doorways.

Salt any other doorways that lead to the outside.

Sprinkle salt along your windowsills and around any hearths.

Say, 'This is my safe space'.

In folklore, it's considered bad luck
to lend salt in case the receiver uses
your salt to curse you at a later date!

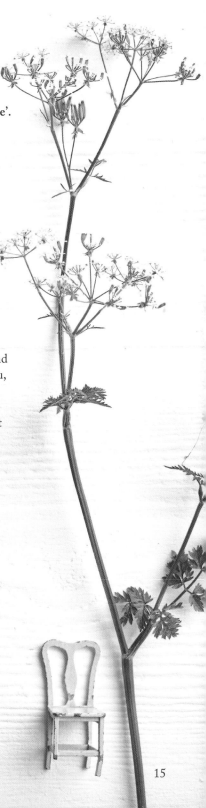

Meringues & Clotted Cream

Magic sometimes calls for ingredients to be combined in a cauldron before a spell can be cast and, for me, recipes hold a similar kind of magical power. They are often made with a clear intention in mind – to soothe or warm, comfort or heal, or to convey care and affection. This simple recipe for fluffy, white meringues is perfect for days when you – or a friend – need to feel a little 'lighter'. The meringues are delicious with fresh fruit and cream – or with cooked apples for an autumnal treat.

Makes 8 meringues

* ★ 3 egg whites
* ★ pinch of salt
* ★ 175g/6oz/1 cup caster sugar
* ★ ½ tsp ground cinnamon
* ★ fresh fruit, to serve
* ★ clotted cream, to serve

Preheat the oven to 140°C/120°C fan/275°F/gas mark 1.

Line two baking trays with baking paper (as the meringue mixture is very sticky).

Whisk the egg whites and salt until the mixture is fairly stiff and fluffy.

Add the sugar very slowly, one tablespoonful at a time, whisking continuously until the mixture is stiff and glossy.

Using two metal spoons, scoop your mixture into 8 mounds – evenly space 4 onto each lined tray.

Sprinkle the cinnamon over the top of the meringues.

Bake for 30–40 minutes until your meringues look crisp and sound hollow when tapped.

Turn off the heat and allow the meringues to cool in the oven with the door slightly ajar. Serve with fruit and cream.

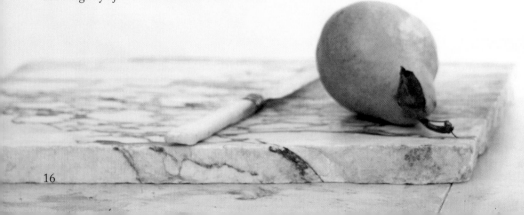

Clotted Cream

Makes approximately 150g/5¼oz of delicious clotted cream

⋆ 1 litre/1¾ pints/4⅓ cups whipping cream or double cream

Pour the cream into a heatproof bowl and place over a saucepan of gently simmering water.

Simmer for 2–3 hours, but don't be tempted to stir it.

Once a thick crust has developed on the top, take the bowl off the heat.

Once cool, cover with a clean tea towel and refrigerate the cream overnight.

Carefully transfer the crust and cream, leaving the liquid behind, into a jar or small bowl, then serve. (Tip: the remaining milk can be used to make delicious scones.)

Leftover cream should be kept in the fridge and will last for about 3–4 days.

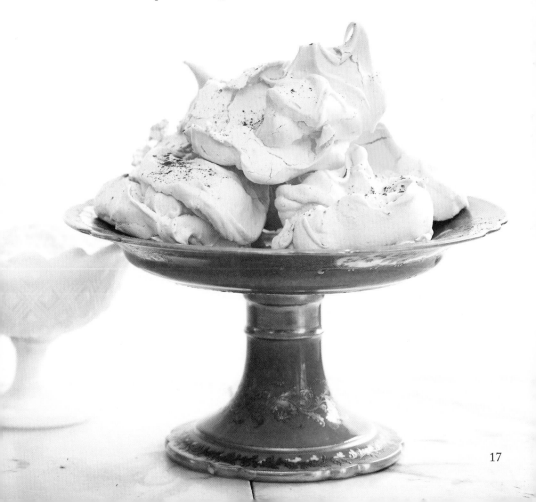

Meadowsweet

Queen of the meadow, meadow wort, meadow queen, dolloff, meadsweet and bridewort

Meadowsweet is a sweet-flavoured, scented herb with frothy white flowers. It loves to grow in damp conditions, particularly in wildflower meadows, marshes and woodlands. This stalwart of nature's medicine cabinet has been recognized for centuries for its therapeutic and magical qualities.

Long prized for its anti-inflammatory properties, it has been used to treat a wide range of ailments, from headaches, indigestion and fever to rheumatism, arthritis and ulcers.

A sacred herb of the ancient Druids, its flowers were laid at ceremonial burial sites. Queen Elizabeth I is said to have walked upon floors strewn with meadowsweet to mask the smell of the Elizabethan court and to ward off infection.

Modern-day Druids use meadowsweet flowers in many rites of passage – including handfasting, marriage and funeral ceremonies, birth celebrations and coming of age and magical rituals.

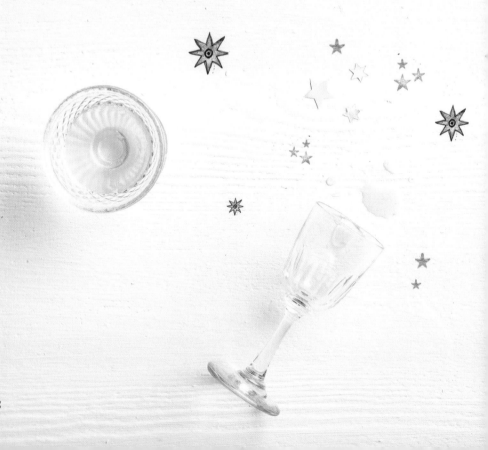

Meadowsweet Cordial

It's easy to make a cleansing, floral cordial with meadowsweet. When kept in the fridge, your cordial should last for 4–6 weeks. It's delicious mixed with water – and with champagne or gin!

Makes about 750ml/1⅓ pints

★ 500g/1lb 2oz/2¾ cups caster sugar, divided into two bowls

★ juice of 2 lemons

★ large bunch of meadowsweet, approximately 60 flower heads

Bring 2 litres/3½ pints/8½ cups water to the boil in a large pan with a lid.

Dissolve half the sugar in the boiling water.

Add the lemon juice, then strip the petals from the flower heads and add to the mixture.

Once simmering, turn off the heat, stir the mixture, pop the lid on and leave to cool in the pan overnight.

Strain the liquid into a jug and discard the petals.

Return the liquid to the pan and add the rest of the sugar.

Bring to the boil and reduce for 5 minutes, then turn off the heat.

While the cordial is hot, pour it carefully into warm, clean, sterilized bottles.

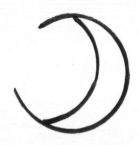

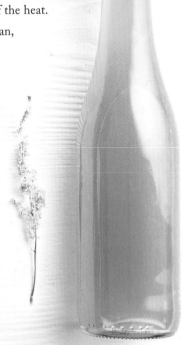

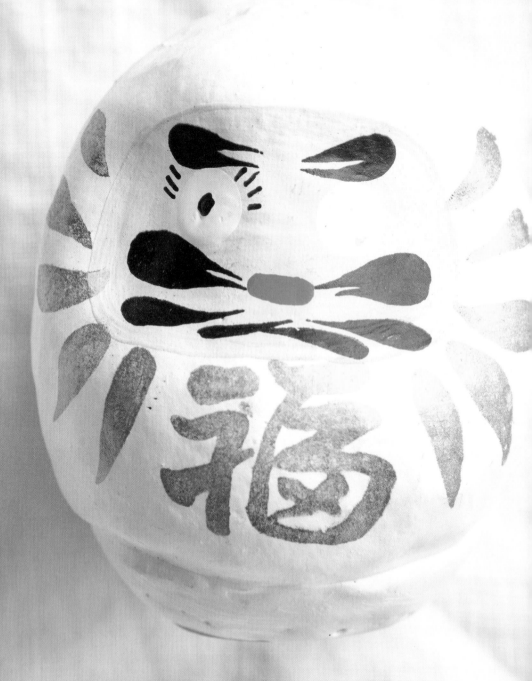

Japanese Daruma

A Daruma is regarded as a talisman of luck and is often given as a gift of encouragement to someone working towards a specific goal. These hollow, papier-mâché figures are modelled after Bodhidharma, the founder of Zen Buddhism in China.

I was given a white Daruma in Japan by a friend, which symbolizes harmony and love. Darumas come in a variety of colours each with their own symbolic meaning. You can choose a Daruma in the colour that reflects the nature of your goal or wish.

WHITE   Harmony & love

YELLOW Protection & security

RED   Good luck & fortune

PINK   Love & romance

VIOLET Health & longevity

GREEN   Beauty & health

BLACK   Wealth & secrets

GOLD   Wealth & prosperity

Initially a Daruma doesn't have eyes. You add one eye when you set your goal or make your wish, and complete the second as your wish or goal is achieved.

Decide on your goal or make a wish.

Draw on one eye.

Focus on your goal or wish.

Draw on the second eye once your goal has been achieved or your wish fulfilled.

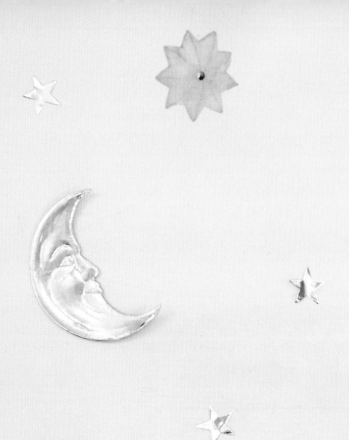

Smoke

Cleansing with the power of smoke is one of my favourite forms of magic. I often burn herbs or incense when making my spells – the smell of smoke helps to create a calm environment in which I can focus on my intention.

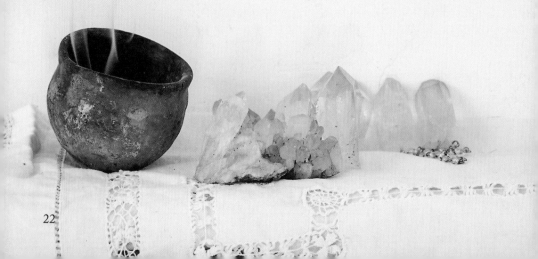

White Sigil

Remembering that the colour white helps us with fresh starts and new beginnings, an intention you could centre your sigil around is...

I AM LIGHT

Breathe.

Write your intention down on paper.

Remove the vowels and any repeated letters...
~~I AM LIGHT~~

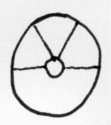

Look at the letters you are left with...
M L G H T

Using the letters that are left, create a symbol on paper – practise a few.

How does that look and feel?

When you are ready, draw your sigil onto a fresh, white candle with a sharp pencil, crayon or pin.

Breathe.

Light your candle.

As it burns, concentrate your intention into the flame.

Keep your mind clear.

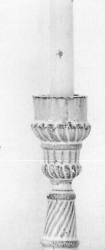

Make sure you keep a note of the sigil in your sigil diary and date it - it's always helpful to look back on your past intentions.

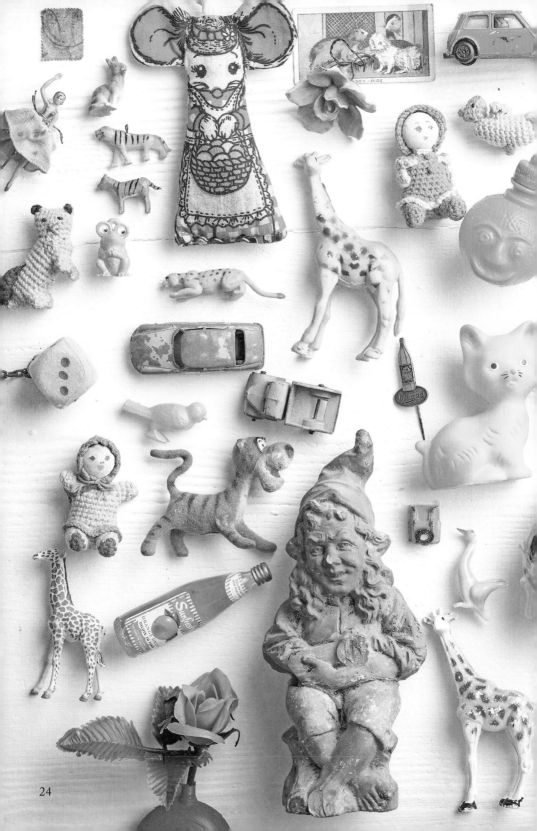

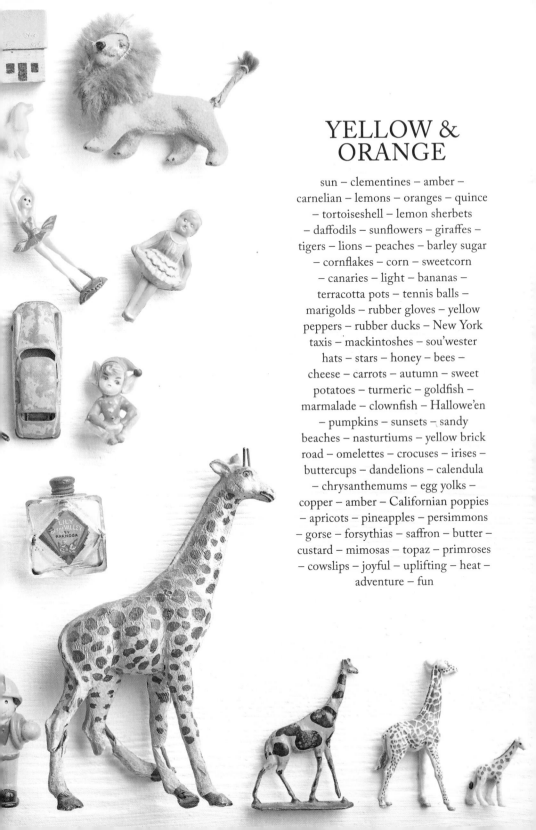

YELLOW & ORANGE

sun – clementines – amber – carnelian – lemons – oranges – quince – tortoiseshell – lemon sherbets – daffodils – sunflowers – giraffes – tigers – lions – peaches – barley sugar – cornflakes – corn – sweetcorn – canaries – light – bananas – terracotta pots – tennis balls – marigolds – rubber gloves – yellow peppers – rubber ducks – New York taxis – mackintoshes – sou'wester hats – stars – honey – bees – cheese – carrots – autumn – sweet potatoes – turmeric – goldfish – marmalade – clownfish – Hallowe'en – pumpkins – sunsets – sandy beaches – nasturtiums – yellow brick road – omelettes – crocuses – irises – buttercups – dandelions – calendula – chrysanthemums – egg yolks – copper – amber – Californian poppies – apricots – pineapples – persimmons – gorse – forsythias – saffron – butter – custard – mimosas – topaz – primroses – cowslips – joyful – uplifting – heat – adventure – fun

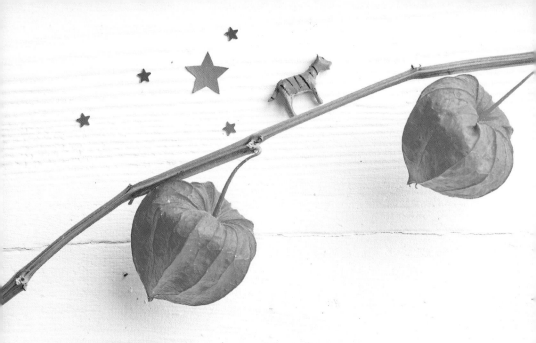

YELLOW & ORANGE

Yellow and orange are the perfect hues to help you make some uplifting, joyous magic. Both yellow and orange have a cheery, playful element to them. They suggest zesty abundance, cocktails at sunset and sun-drenched cornfields. These colours can conjure up feelings of heat, adventure and fun, perfect for when you may need an energy boost.

Of course, both colours have a strong association with the sun – which ancient civilizations revered, as we do today, as the source of life. Sunshine on our faces, as well as being a pleasure, also helps us to create vitamin D. As well as keeping our bones, teeth and muscles healthy, vitamin D can help us feel brighter, while the sun is known to help boost the metabolism.

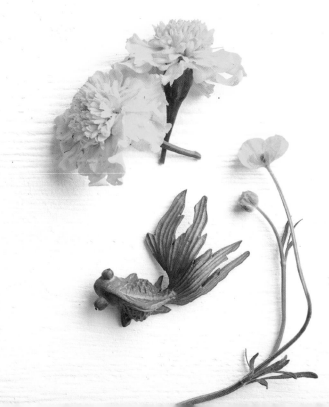

Yellow and orange can also be relied upon to attract prosperity. During Chinese New Year celebrations, tangerines and oranges are eaten to attract good luck and happiness. Eating an orange or drinking lemon tea can give you a zingy, fresh feeling.

altar

flower: marigold, sunflower
crystals & gems: tiger's eye, citrine, topaz
element: fire

IN CHINESE TRADITION, GOLDFISH SYMBOLIZE GOOD FORTUNE

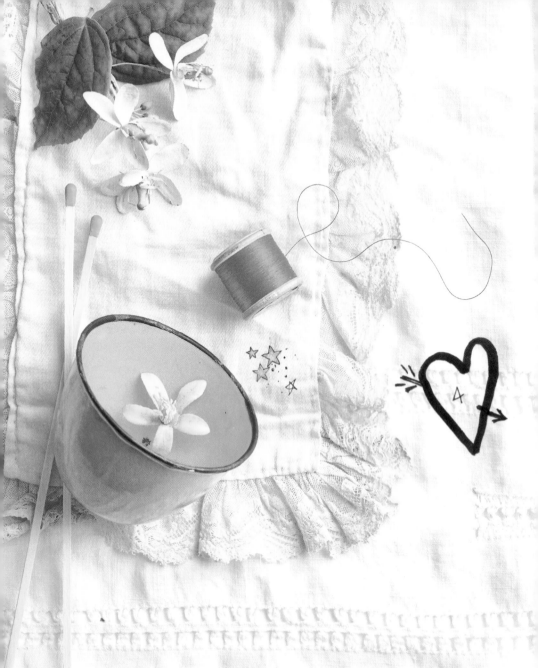

The divinely scented orange blossom flower became a popular feature in bridal garlands in the Victorian era – Queen Victoria wore a headdress made from the flowers and her wedding dress was trimmed with blossom and lace. Orange blossom flowers can be used to make a strong love spell.

Orange Blossom Love Spell

This love spell can help strengthen your ties to a person you are in a relationship with. Focus on your feelings for that person as you settle on your intention for this spell. Before you begin, you'll need a fireproof bowl and a well-ventilated room.

Cast your spell

* 3 or 4 dried orange blossom flowers
* your true love's name written on a small piece of paper
* your name written on a small piece of paper
* match
* handkerchief and orange thread

Breathe.

Focus on your feelings for your true love.

Burn the dried flowers and names in a fireproof bowl.

Allow the ashes to cool.

Breathe.

Place them in a handkerchief.

Tie the cloth with orange thread.

If you need to release this spell, pour the ashes into running water and focus on letting your feelings go.

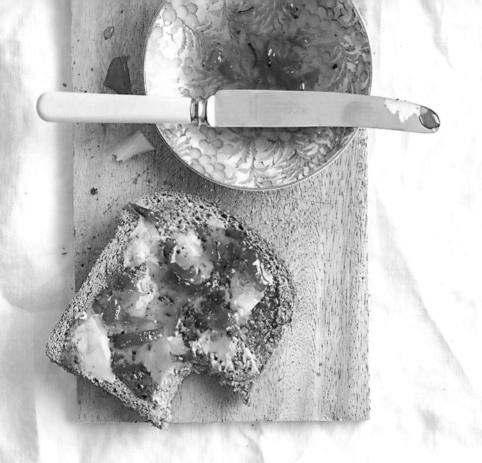

Marmalade

Seville oranges are steeped in ancient folklore. The Roman god Hercules was said to have been sent on a quest to find them. The oil from the orange blossom peel can be used to create a scented elixir with healing and restorative powers. This bittersweet preserve is sure to bring a warm smile, whatever the weather. It's delicious on toast, with porridge and as a filling in cakes. A certain bear is said to love a marmalade sandwich – who doesn't?

Place the whole oranges and lemon juice into a large saucepan.

Cover with 2.5 litres/4½ pints/generous 10 cups water and simmer for 2 hours over a low heat.

Warm the sugar for about 1 hour in a very low oven. Remove from the oven and set aside.

Remove the pan from the heat. Strain the liquid into a jug and tip the oranges into a bowl.

Return the cooking liquid to the pan.

Carefully scoop the flesh out of the oranges and add to the pan. Keep the peel to one side.

Boil the orange pulp and strained cooking liquid for 8–10 minutes.

Remove the pan from the heat. Strain the liquid into a bowl, pressing with a wooden spoon to get all of the juice through.

Pour the liquid back into the saucepan.

Slice the peel into small thin strips.

Add the peel and the warmed sugar to the pan with the cooking liquid.

Stir gently over a low heat for 10 minutes to allow the sugar to dissolve.

Bring to the boil, allowing your mixture to bubble rapidly for 18–30 minutes until the setting point is reached. The best way to test this is to use a jam thermometer – bring the marmalade to 105°C/222°F.

Skim any scum from the top of your mixture – adding a knob of butter to the surface and stirring it in gently can help to dispel any remaining cloudiness.

Leave to cool for 20 minutes, then pour carefully into warm, clean, sterilized jars, and label. Leave to cool completely, then tightly seal and store in a cool, dry place. Once opened, keep the marmalade in the fridge and use within 3–4 weeks.

Fills about 8 jam jars

* ★ 1.3kg/3lb Seville oranges
* ★ juice of 3 small lemons
* ★ 2kg/4½lb/10 cups granulated sugar
* ★ 1 tsp salted butter

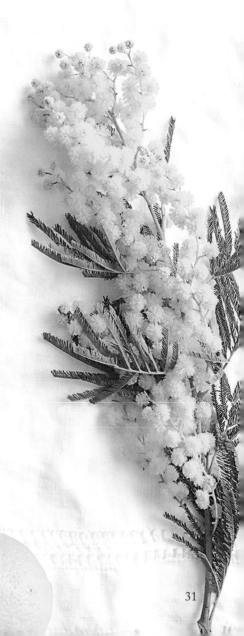

Amber

Amber is fossilized tree resin, revered since Neolithic times. Beautiful and curious, amber is most valuable when it contains insects – caught in the resin as it formed millions of years before. Amber can have great clarity, patterns, swirls and even stripes.

Amber has been used for centuries across Europe as a soothing gem for children and is thought to offer protection and relieve anxiety.

Children were often gifted amber necklaces at birth and mothers are awarded their 'tiger stripe' stretch marks for their courage and bravery. Amber acts as a natural analgesic when worn against the skin as beads.

Faceted amber became hugely popular in Georgian and Victorian times, especially for earrings as it is incredibly light to wear.

Search for old vintage amber beads at markets – as well as being kinder to the environment, it's a joyful treasure hunt.

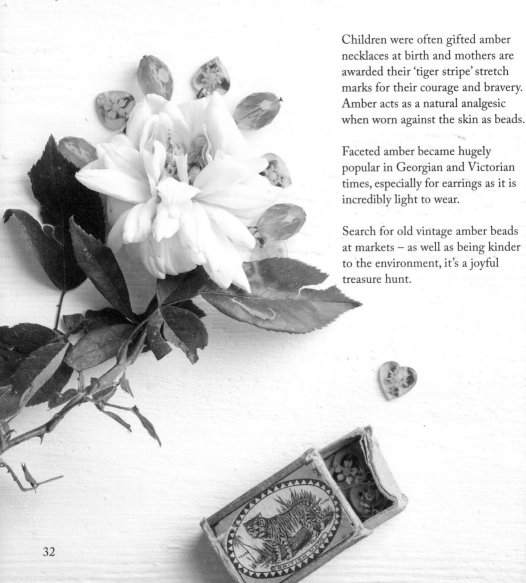

The Tyger

By William Blake

Tyger Tyger, burning bright,
In the forests of the night;
What immortal hand or eye,
Could frame thy fearful symmetry?

In what distant deeps or skies.
Burnt the fire of thine eyes?
On what wings dare he aspire?
What the hand, dare seize the fire?

And what shoulder, & what art,
Could twist the sinews of thy heart?
And when thy heart began to beat,
What dread hand? & what dread feet?

What the hammer? what the chain,
In what furnace was thy brain?
What the anvil? what dread grasp,
Dare its deadly terrors clasp!

When the stars threw down their spears
And water'd heaven with their tears:
Did he smile his work to see?
Did he who made the Lamb make thee?

Tyger Tyger burning bright,
In the forests of the night:
What immortal hand or eye,
Dare frame thy fearful symmetry?

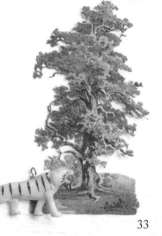

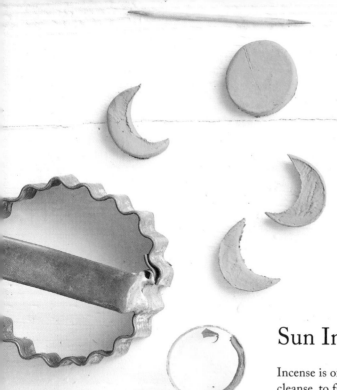

Sun Incense Holder

Incense is often used for spiritual rituals: to cleanse, to fragrance a space, to set a mood, and to create an ethereal and meditative moment for reflection. Lighting incense makes the statement that you are making space to focus on your personal, magical work.

This simple incense stick holder is made from terracotta air-drying clay. Don't worry if you don't have any biscuit cutters, you can use the rim of a glass instead. You could make the holder in the shape of a star, square, pentagram or moon, but I wanted a simple sun to add brightness and energy to my intentions.

* air-drying clay
* rolling pin
* 6cm/2½in round fluted biscuit cutter, or a drinking glass
* cutlery for shaping and piercing
* packet of wooden cocktail sticks
* small circle of foil

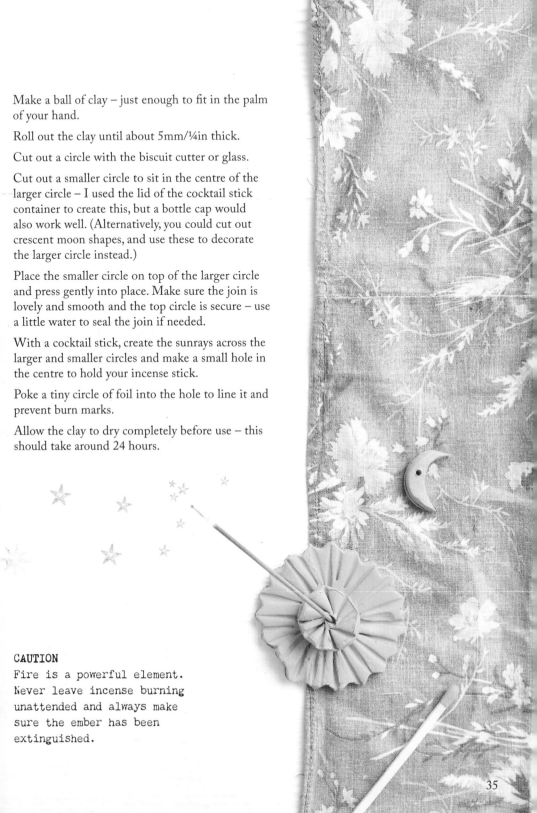

Make a ball of clay – just enough to fit in the palm of your hand.

Roll out the clay until about 5mm/¼in thick.

Cut out a circle with the biscuit cutter or glass.

Cut out a smaller circle to sit in the centre of the larger circle – I used the lid of the cocktail stick container to create this, but a bottle cap would also work well. (Alternatively, you could cut out crescent moon shapes, and use these to decorate the larger circle instead.)

Place the smaller circle on top of the larger circle and press gently into place. Make sure the join is lovely and smooth and the top circle is secure – use a little water to seal the join if needed.

With a cocktail stick, create the sunrays across the larger and smaller circles and make a small hole in the centre to hold your incense stick.

Poke a tiny circle of foil into the hole to line it and prevent burn marks.

Allow the clay to dry completely before use – this should take around 24 hours.

CAUTION
Fire is a powerful element. Never leave incense burning unattended and always make sure the ember has been extinguished.

35

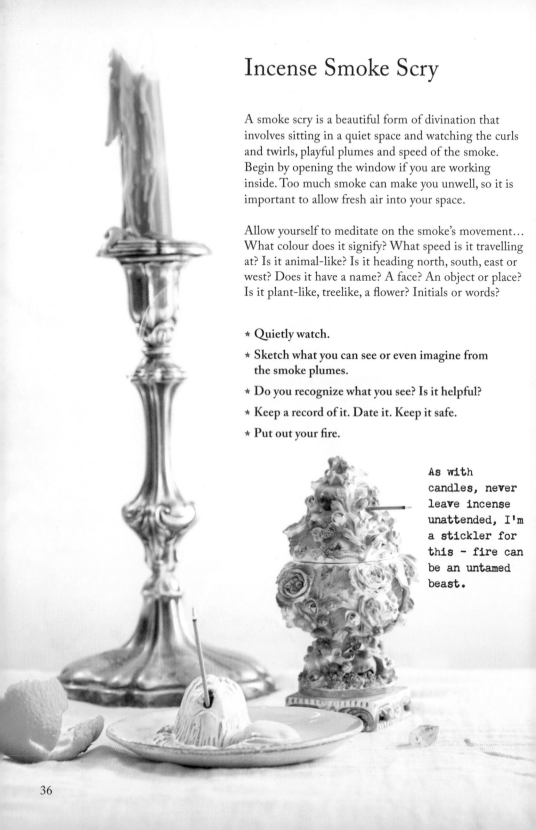

Incense Smoke Scry

A smoke scry is a beautiful form of divination that involves sitting in a quiet space and watching the curls and twirls, playful plumes and speed of the smoke. Begin by opening the window if you are working inside. Too much smoke can make you unwell, so it is important to allow fresh air into your space.

Allow yourself to meditate on the smoke's movement... What colour does it signify? What speed is it travelling at? Is it animal-like? Is it heading north, south, east or west? Does it have a name? A face? An object or place? Is it plant-like, treelike, a flower? Initials or words?

* Quietly watch.
* Sketch what you can see or even imagine from the smoke plumes.
* Do you recognize what you see? Is it helpful?
* Keep a record of it. Date it. Keep it safe.
* Put out your fire.

As with candles, never leave incense unattended, I'm a stickler for this - fire can be an untamed beast.

Yellow & Orange Sigil

Sometime we can drift, sleepwalking under a sort of cloud – as if a sludgy inactive, sad blanket is covering us. You can use colour to shake this feeling off, to take a big breath and reignite your energy and fire. Be inspired by the zesty, energetic, fire qualities of these citrus colours and perhaps settle on a statement or intention of fun, joy or adventure. Using orange or yellow crayons is the perfect way to activate intentions strengthened by these colours.

I AM AWAKE
Remove the vowels and any repeated letters...

~~I AM AWAKE~~

Look at the letters you are left with…

MWK

Play with the letters.

Breathe.

Allow yourself some time to settle.

Focus on your desire.

Breathe.

Draw out your sigil on paper.

Place your paper in a fireproof bowl and light it.

As your sigil burns, allow your energy to rise.

Wide awake.

Make sure your ashes and candle are extinguished.

Forest Bathing

Connecting to nature and our old ancient ways is one of the best ways to begin your magical journey. Forest bathing has gained popularity as a beneficial pastime, particularly in Japan where it is known as *shinrin-yoku*. Walking amongst trees in a wood, a forest or even in your local city park will help you unwind.

Breathe.

Look at the yellow sunshine filtering through the trees, allow the light to play on your face.

Allow tension and stress to slip away as you walk.

Shake the energy from your fingertips.

Sit with your back against a tree.

Imagine the tree's roots beneath you, under the very soil you are sitting on, supporting you as you sit, connected deep into the earth's core.

Relax.

Watch the sunset, knowing you have had a good day.

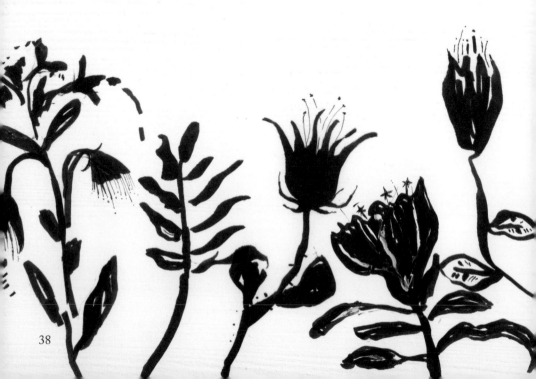

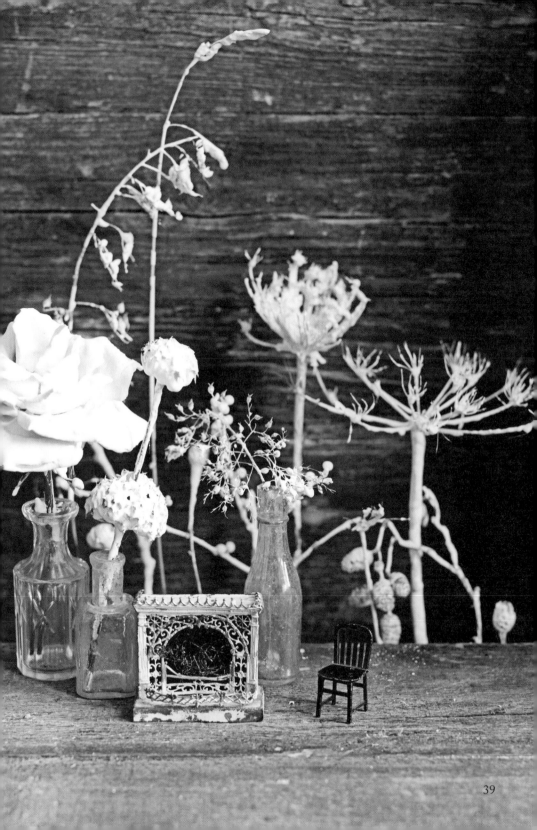

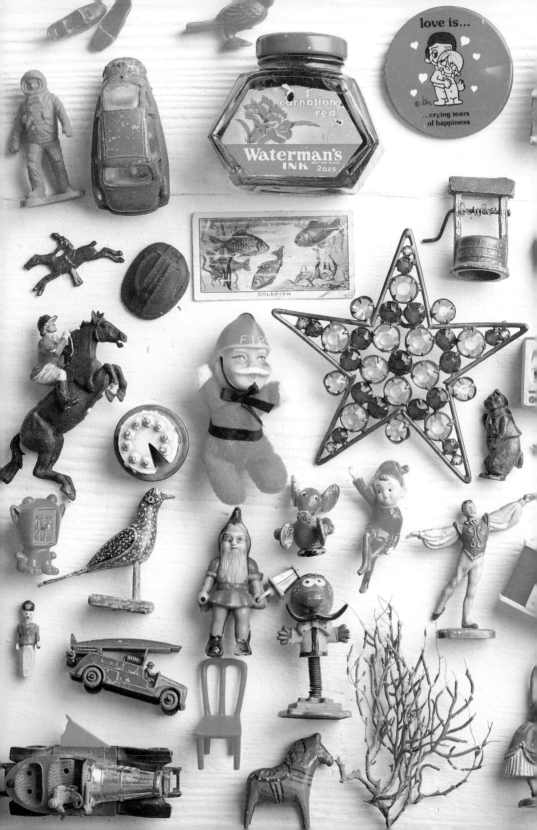

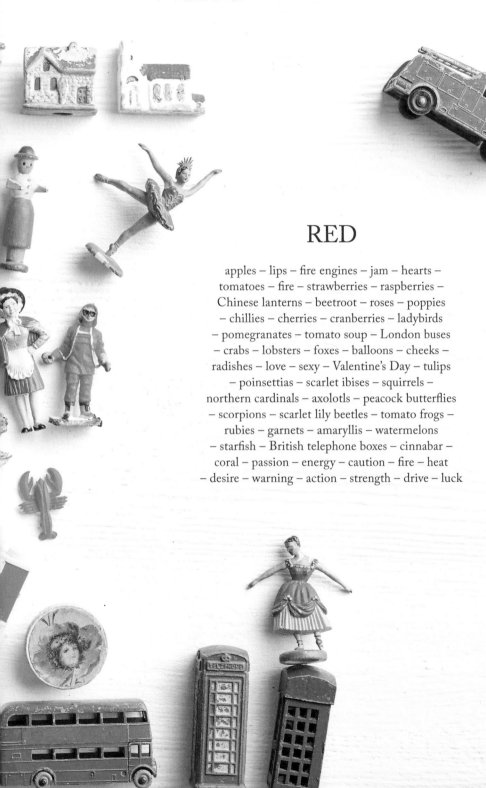

RED

apples – lips – fire engines – jam – hearts –
tomatoes – fire – strawberries – raspberries –
Chinese lanterns – beetroot – roses – poppies
– chillies – cherries – cranberries – ladybirds
– pomegranates – tomato soup – London buses
– crabs – lobsters – foxes – balloons – cheeks –
radishes – love – sexy – Valentine's Day – tulips
– poinsettias – scarlet ibises – squirrels –
northern cardinals – axolotls – peacock butterflies
– scorpions – scarlet lily beetles – tomato frogs –
rubies – garnets – amaryllis – watermelons
– starfish – British telephone boxes – cinnabar –
coral – passion – energy – caution – fire – heat
– desire – warning – action – strength – drive – luck

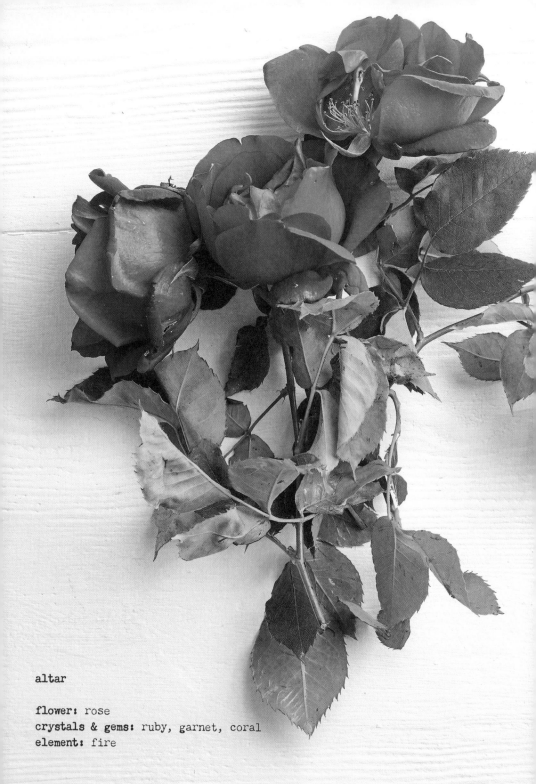

altar

flower: rose
crystals & gems: ruby, garnet, coral
element: fire

42

RED

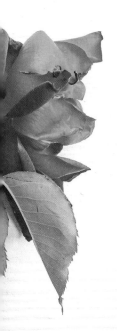

Red is a hugely powerful, sexy, fiery colour. The shade evokes a range of feelings from love, lust and desire to heated emotion and anger (flushed, furious cheeks). Think seductive, secret Valentine, a fairy-tale forest of ruby red roses, the scarlet cloak of Little Red Riding Hood and the red, red mouth of the wolf.

Red shades are perfect when you are in need of passion, drive, or a change of direction and can fill you with an energetic desire to 'act now'. Red is also a warning colour so make your intentions and wishes very precise.

Red can also provide a wonderful subliminal protection against negativity. Try wearing something red or a red thread tied on your wrist when you need courage and bravery. Red is the colour of our heart, our blood and core, so use the power of red when you need to stand tall and be strong.

Red symbolizes joy and good fortune across the world. The Lunar New Year is celebrated in China with red lanterns and garland streamers, while children are gifted red envelopes containing money. Chinese brides are often wed in red. Wearing red is said to terrify and protect you from the fearsome dragon monster, Nian, who is said to visit on the Lunar New Year's Eve.

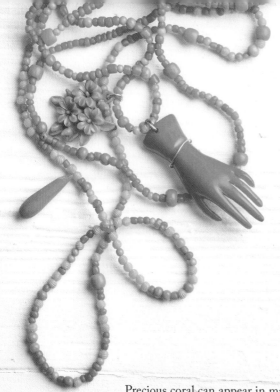

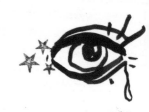

Coral

My favourite protective stone.

Red coral, in ancient European folklore, was considered a gift from the gods and revered as magical tokens from the sea if found upon a beach. There are records that say that coral was ground and used as an ingredient for an incense commonly known as 'Venus incense' in the sixteenth century in Italy. This incense was widely believed to attract sexual passion. A love spell indeed.

Precious coral can appear in many hues: deep blood reds, glowing oranges or the most beautiful palest pinks (known as angel skin coral).

Coral was traditionally given as a gift of protection, along with amber, to protect and nurture a child from harm. Polished coral handles for Victorian silver rattles are quite often found in museum collections. The wonderful Foundling Museum in London, which explores the history of the Foundling Hospital (the UK's first children's charity), has a heartbreaking collection of eighteenth-century 'tokens': when a mother had to leave her baby in the care of the hospital, she left behind a 'token' for her child so she could recognize and be reunited with them if her fortunes changed. The tokens in the collection include fragments of fabric, drawings, buttons, a patch of petticoat, charms and, memorably, a single coral bead.

It's important to remember that our coral reefs are under threat and need to be protected, so only ever repurpose vintage coral jewellery for spell work.

I recommend sewing a single vintage bead inside your coat for protection.

Sweetheart Spell

The desire to receive or send love is as old as the hills and often the reason many are drawn towards magic. It's important to cast this spell to attract a particular kind of love rather than attract a specific someone. Visualize the type of person you would like to love and to love you – don't be vague. Take time to be sure of your intention.

Always remember to make your intention honourable

You are looking for a true love

NEVER coerce another

NEVER steal another's love

* red candle
* paper
* red pen
* red thread

Light the candle.

Breathe.

Focus on the smoke rising.

When ready, write the qualities of your true love on the piece of paper.

Roll it up.

Tie with red thread.

Carefully seal the knot with candle wax.

Sometimes, as time goes on, what we have craved and wished for has either become real or is no longer wanted. If a spell is no longer relevant to you, burn your spell in a fireproof bowl, completely, then release the ashes into running water such as a river, the sea or under a running tap is just fine.

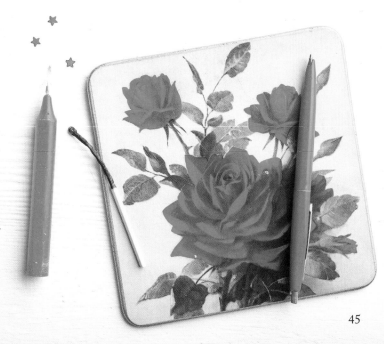

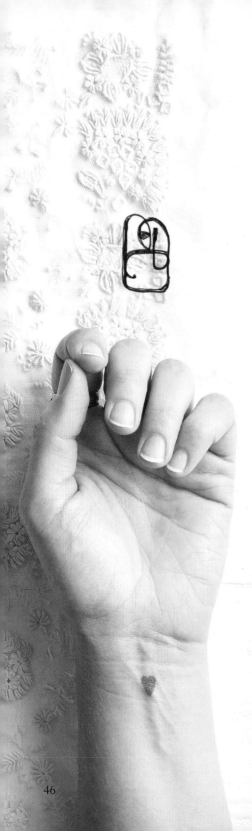

Red Sigil

Red is a powerful colour to help you manifest your intentions. Use this colour to activate strong, deep, fiery and energetic magic. Romantic, sensual and sexual, red can also fire things up a little. As with all magic, make sure you are clear about what you are asking for.

A simple sigil could be designed from a statement such as...

I ATTRACT LOVE

Remove all the vowels and repeated letters...
I̶ A̶T̶T̶R̶A̶C̶T̶ L̶O̶V̶E̶

Look at the letters you are left with...
T R C L V

Play with your letters to form a symbol. How does that feel? Need a flourish? Perhaps add a heart and arrow.

When you feel your symbol is right for you, draw out your sigil on some paper and pop it in your locket, pocket or drawer.

Make a note of your sigil and date it.

Try drawing your symbol on your wrist in red, or perhaps draw a heart to give you focus and strengthen your magic.

Red Chilli Oil

This delicious spiced oil can be drizzled over pizza and pasta dishes, and is great in salad dressings. Perfect for when you want to add a little heat!

Makes about 300ml/10½fl oz

* 1 heaped tbsp chilli flakes
* 1 heaped tbsp chilli powder
* 300ml/10½fl oz/1¼ cups olive oil
* 5 star anise
* 1 cinnamon stick
* 1 tbsp Szechuan peppercorns
* 1 tbsp cardamom pods
* 3 bay leaves

Add the chilli flakes and powder to a warm, clean, sterilized glass jar.

Heat the oil gently in a saucepan.

Toast the remaining spices and bay leaves in a dry frying pan over a gentle heat so that the fragrance is released and the spices begin to smoke very gently. Be careful not to burn them.

Carefully add the toasted spices and bay leaves to the warm oil and allow the oil to simmer for 5 minutes over a low heat.

Slowly strain the oil into the jar and stir with a metal spoon to combine.

Add a few of the leftover spices to the jar.

Allow to cool completely, then tightly seal. Store in an cool, dry place and use within a month.

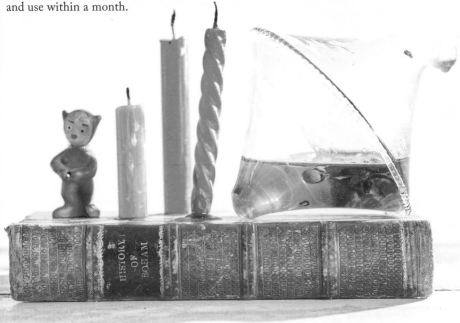

Red Berry Compote

Any soft fruit can be used for this recipe, which is a lovely way to use up fruit that is on the turn. This compote is best served warm, but it's delicious with granola too – just leave the compote to cool completely and chill it before serving.

Serves 10

* 175g/6oz raspberries
* 175g/6oz strawberries
* 175g/6oz redcurrants
* 175g/6oz blackberries
* 3 peaches, stones removed
* 3 apricots, stones removed
* 50g/1¾oz/heaped ¼ cup caster sugar, or more to taste
* ice cream or yogurt, to serve

Preheat the oven to 180°C/160°C fan/350°F/gas mark 4.

Slice the fruit and transfer it to a large ovenproof dish.

Stir in the sugar.

Cover with foil and cook for approximately 1 hour until cooked through and soft.

Remove from the oven, carefully remove the foil and check – if the mixture looks a little dry, add a small amount of water.

Cook, uncovered, for a further 20 minutes or until all the fruit has softened – the juices will have oozed and formed a delicious compote.

Serve warm with vanilla ice cream or chilled plain yogurt.

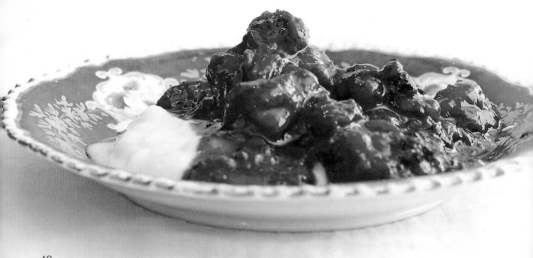

Lucky Red Wrist Ribbon

As we know, red is a colour of passion, action, strength, love and drive.
Use this colour to help you reach for the stars.

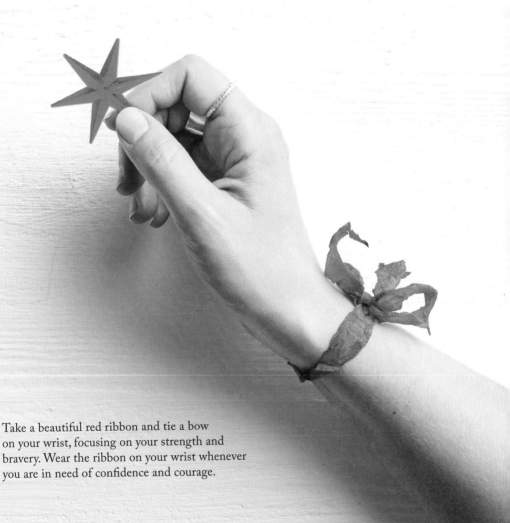

Take a beautiful red ribbon and tie a bow
on your wrist, focusing on your strength and
bravery. Wear the ribbon on your wrist whenever
you are in need of confidence and courage.

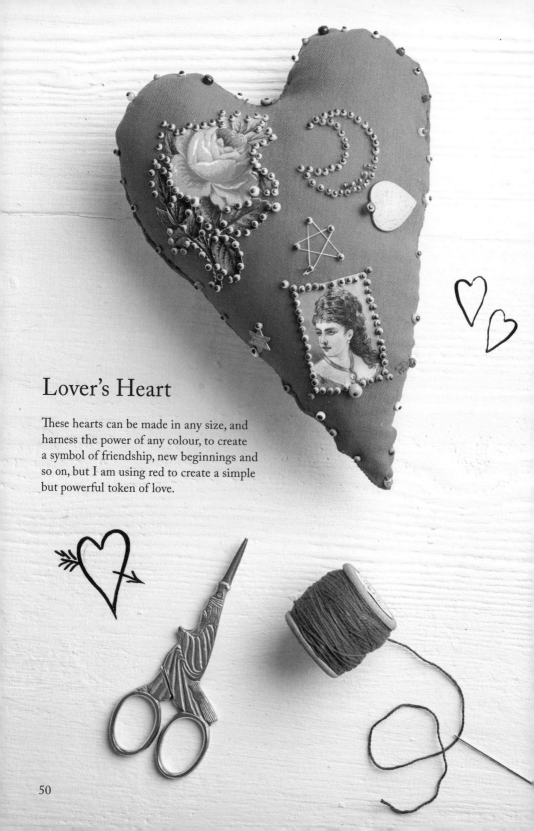

Lover's Heart

These hearts can be made in any size, and harness the power of any colour, to create a symbol of friendship, new beginnings and so on, but I am using red to create a simple but powerful token of love.

* scissors
* paper and pencil
* 2 pieces of red fabric, each about 20cm x 20cm/8in x 8in
* pins, metal-ended

* coloured silk and cotton threads
* needle
* approx. 600g/1lb 5oz play sand
* paper decorations (see below for ideas)
* selection of beads and charms

Make a paper stencil of a heart shape that fits comfortably within the measurements of your fabric – you could choose the traditional valentine shape or witch's heart shape, where the tail twists to one side (see page 139).

Pin around the two pieces of fabric, with the right sides together.

Pin the heart stencil on top and cut around the shape.

Pin around the fabric hearts, with the right sides together.

Sew all the way around your heart with backstitch to prevent the sand used to fill the heart from escaping, leaving a gap of around 2.5cm/1in unsewn. Remove the pins.

Turn the heart inside out.

Fill your heart with sand until it feels quite firm.

Tuck in the unsewn edges and stitch them firmly in place.

Start by decorating the centre of your token. Would you like to use a photo of your true love? Or a picture of a friend, family member or pet? You could also use sigils or magical symbols, flowers, initials… whatever feels right.

To secure your photo, take a pin and thread a bead on the end, push it down firmly through the paper and into the sand to secure the first corner of your picture in place. (This is why the heart needs to be packed tightly.)

Continue to frame the picture with beaded pins to fix it in place. Maybe alternate your bead colours.

Create a pattern around the edges of your heart with more beaded pins.

You could also use embroidery thread and pins to create patterns and symbols, add fringing, or pin lucky charms to your heart.

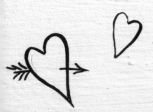

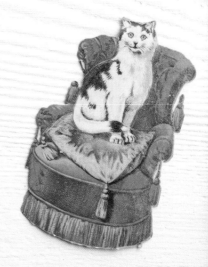

The Song of Wandering Aengus

By William Butler Yeats

I went out to the hazel wood,
Because a fire was in my head,
And cut and peeled a hazel wand,
And hooked a berry to a thread;
And when white moths were on the wing,
And moth-like stars were flickering out,
I dropped the berry in a stream
And caught a little silver trout.

When I had laid it on the floor
I went to blow the fire a-flame,
But something rustled on the floor,
And someone called me by my name:
It had become a glimmering girl
With apple blossom in her hair
Who called me by my name and ran
And faded through the brightening air.

Though I am old with wandering
Through hollow lands and hilly lands,
I will find out where she has gone,
And kiss her lips and take her hands;
And walk among long dappled grass,
And pluck till time and times are done,
The silver apples of the moon,
The golden apples of the sun.

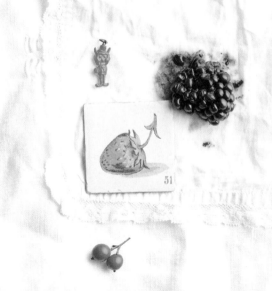

THE BLACKBERRY

A legend tells of the blackberry glowing red as a
coal until Lucifer, thrown from Heaven landed upon
the bush and instantly rendered the fruit black.

Blackberry leaves, stems and thorns can all be
used in potions - especially for portal and altar
blessings. Try using a blackberry stem in a wreath
as a protective home charm.

Redcurrants, strawberries
and raspberries are a sign
of warmer days to come.

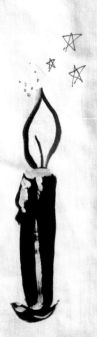

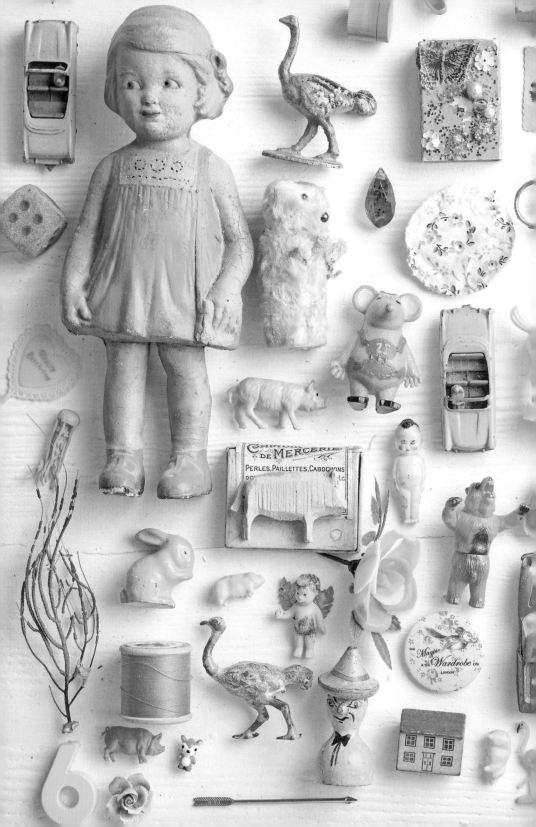

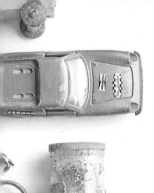

PINK

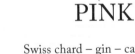

Swiss chard – gin – candy floss –
macarons – cherry blossom – Sakura
– rose water – sea anemones – rose-
breasted cockatoos – marshmallows
– sugared almonds – tutus – blushes
– cats' tongues – bubble gum – seashells
– prawn cocktails – flamingos – cold
noses – peonies – sweet peas – peaches
– foxgloves – Turkish delight – rhubarb –
petal-scattered sheets – roseate spoonbills
– blancmange – Himalayan salt – pink
wafer biscuits – puppies' tummies – good
witches – fairy tales – fairies and the fey
– enchantment – gentleness – laughter
– calmness – youthful – childlike –
tender – kindness – intuition – comfort
– emotional – romantic – peaceful –
healing – friendship – relaxing

PINK

Pink is a colour of love and romance, intuition and serenity, kindness and comfort. Think romance novels and rose petals scattered over bed sheets, enchanting tales of the fey, and fairy cakes covered with pink icing and sprinkles.

In Japan, pink is associated with Sakura, the cherry and plum blossom season. The blooming period symbolizes the arrival of spring, hope, beauty, new life and also, beautifully, acceptance of the fragility of life as the blossoms fall. Sakura season is celebrated by the ritual of Hanami (flower viewing), an ancient Japanese custom of enjoying the delicacy and fleeting nature of the flowers.

Pink can help you to 'melt' – to relax and release pent-up anger, fear, stress or anxiety. It can help make your space become more comforting, safe and relaxing and will strengthen intentions centred around friendship, goodwill and affection. Rose quartz is the perfect crystal to aid your intuition and comfort your soul.

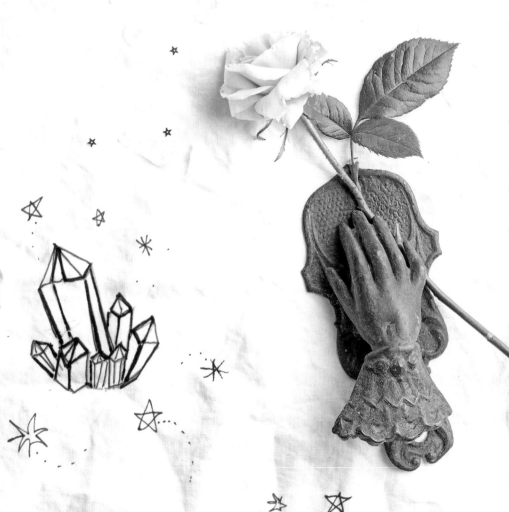

altar

flower: pink carnation
crystals & gems: rose quartz, opal
element: fire

Valentine Chocolate

Chocolate is a well-known gift for friends, kin and, in particular, lovers. It contains phenylethylamine – the chemical our brains produce when we are in love. Chocolate has been scientifically proven to increase feelings of affection and boost libido... what's not to love?

* 300g/10½oz white chocolate
* 150g/5¼oz milk chocolate
* 150g/5¼oz plain chocolate

* pinch of sea salt
* sprinkles
* edible flowers

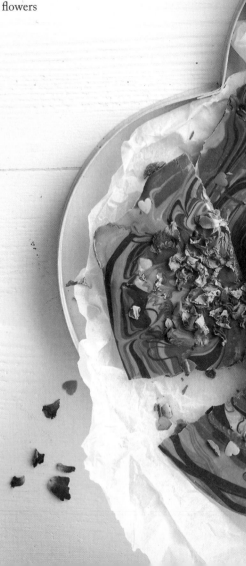

Break the chocolate into squares.

Place a heatproof bowl on top of a pan of gently simmering water – the bowl should sit snugly in the pan but not touch the water.

Add the squares of white chocolate and stir until melted.

Place a second bowl on top of a second pan of gently simmering water, add the milk and plain chocolate squares and leave to melt without stirring.

Pour the melted white chocolate onto a lined baking tray, about 25 x 30cm/10 x 12in.

Slowly pour the milk and plain chocolate mixture into the melted white chocolate and use a fork to gently marble them together.

Adorn the top with sprinkles and edible flowers.

Chill in the fridge for 30 minutes until the chocolate has set.

Break the chocolate into pieces, and transfer to a box or bag.

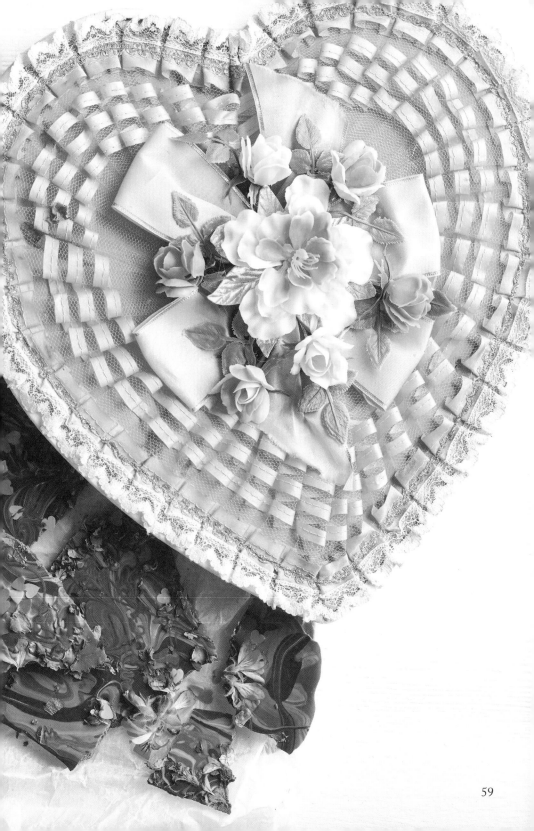

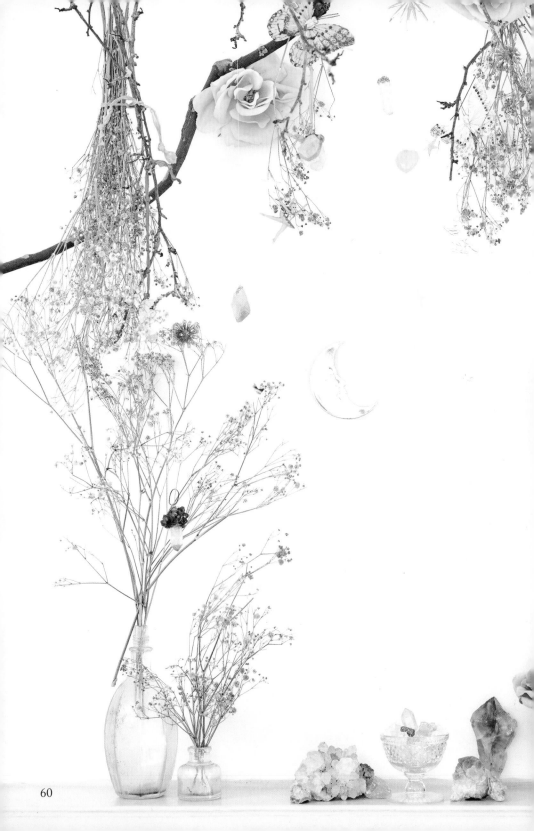

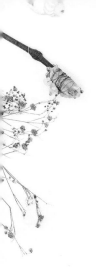

Crystal Grotto

This is a pretty and magical make.
It could decorate an altar, mantelpiece,
windowsill or shelf, and be placed anywhere
in the house. Use this space for spell work.

* fallen branch and a selection of twigs

* wire and cotton thread

* crystals

* paper tape

* eco-friendly glitter

* glue stick

* fripperies that attract you, such as stars, charms, feathers, flowers, jewels and shells

* ribbons

* scissors

Trim your branch as desired and fasten your twigs together with wire to create a frame that is sturdy enough to hang your crystals and fripperies from. Secure the branch in your desired place.

Prepare your crystals by wrapping wire two or three times around the top of each one, securing the wire in place with a little paper tape. If you like you can decorate your tape with glitter using the glue stick.

Thread a piece of cotton through the top of the wire and attach to the twigs so your crystals hang down.

Repeat with as many crystals and fripperies as you like... you may have to add more twigs as you go.

When you are happy, clean your crystal grotto of any negativity – use a sprinkle of salt to cleanse your space (see page 15).

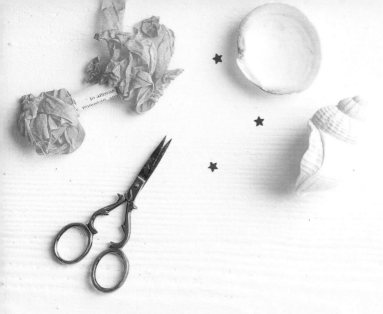

Witches' Knots

Knotting is an ancient form of magic I have practised all my life and it wasn't until I was an adult that I realized it had a name and others did it too. I would often knot threads in patterns and, with a nod of my head, I would tie a wish.

There is the old adage of tying a knot into a handkerchief to remind you of something that must not be forgotten. This magic is not for that which has been forgotten necessarily, but is useful for spells that require intense concentration, intensity and thought. Perhaps a spell regarding a life change, moving house, a shift in relationships or a big event.

When beginning your spell, create a safe space for yourself to work and clear any negative energy with some salt (see page 14). Sometimes just a word can be enough for a spell – working almost as a chant running through your mind as you knot – representing what you have, what you need or perhaps what you desire. Here are a few examples: ABUNDANCE, PLENTY, LOVE, CLARITY and STRENGTH.

You can use rope, thread, cotton or even hair for knot magic. Additional talismans such as feathers or shells, inscribed with words to reinforce your intentions, can be woven into your knots. These are sometimes known as Witches' Ladders.

For this spell, we are using ribbons.

By knot of 1, my spell's begun

By knot of 2, my spell comes true

By knot of 3, it comes to be

By knot of 4, this power I store

By knot of 5, this spell contrive

By knot of 6, this spell I fix

By knot of 7, by earth and heaven

By knot of 8, my will be fate

By knot of 9, what's done is mine

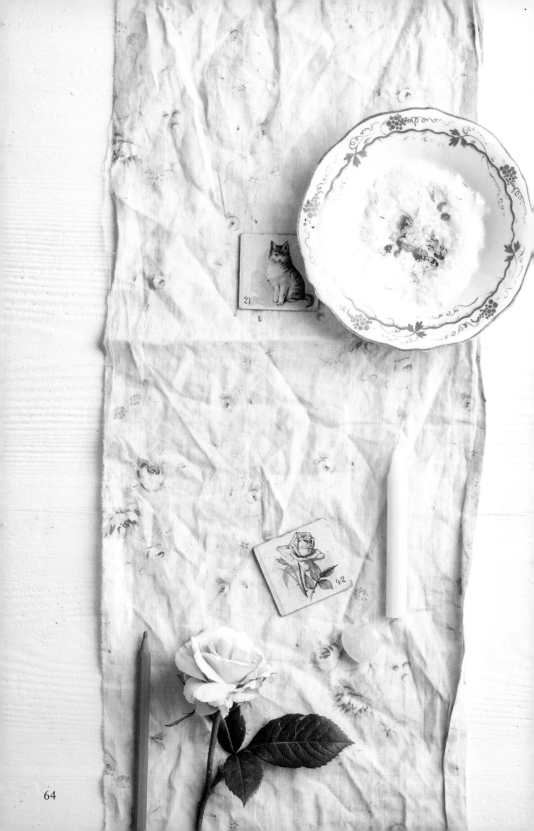

Pink Sigil

Pink, the colour of love and friendship, is the perfect colour
to support intentions focused on releasing pent-up emotions.
Let's try a simple sigil – what will your intention be?

Breathe.

Write your intention down on paper...

I AM RELAXED

Remove all the vowels and repeated letters...

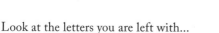

Look at the letters you are left with...

M R L X D

Feel your tension slip away as you breathe deeply and play the
letters into your sigil.

Phew, that's a relief.

Now consider how to activate your pink sigil. What would
feel most comfortable? Try lighting a fresh pink candle.
Alternatively, try taking a small saucer and sprinkling some
salt upon it. Gently, let your finger make your sigil shape in
the salt. If that feels good, relax and enjoy, perhaps keep this
salt with its sigil energy. Remember to make a note of your
sigil as the shapes will fold back into the salt once again.

If it didn't feel good to activate your sigil this way, then wash
the salt away and try again using a different method (see pages
8–9). Again, there are no rules and no single formula.

Friendship Jar Spell

A meaningful gift at the right time is possibly the kindest thing ever. When selecting and combining the ingredients for this friendship charm, concentrate on the loving aspects of your relationship – how much you value the person this spell is intended for and how dear they are to you. Maybe light a pink candle and listen to music or hum a song that means something to you both as you make your jar.

INGREDIENTS

Salt	Cleansing
Rose petals	Love and protection, romance
Rose quartz	Intuition, compassion and empathy
Cinnamon stick	Energy
Geranium leaves or petals	Happiness, laughter
Honeysuckle petals	Stability

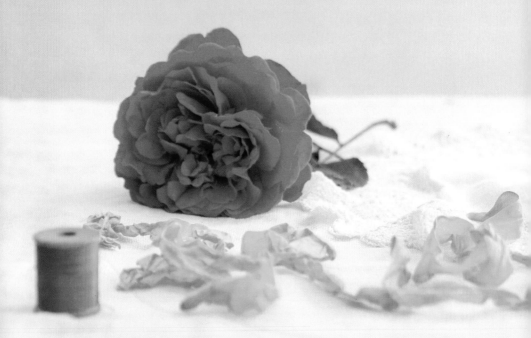

* your choice of ingredients
* small jar with a lid
* few drops of rose oil, optional
* paper and pen
* pink ribbon or thread

Choose the ingredients that will support your friendship and combine them in the jar. Add a few drops of rose oil, if you like.

Write the initials of your friend on a piece of paper and add this to the jar.

Seal the jar tightly with a lid.

Tie the pink ribbon or thread around the lid.

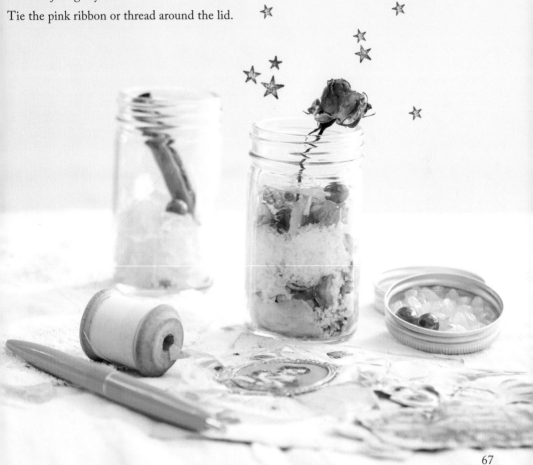

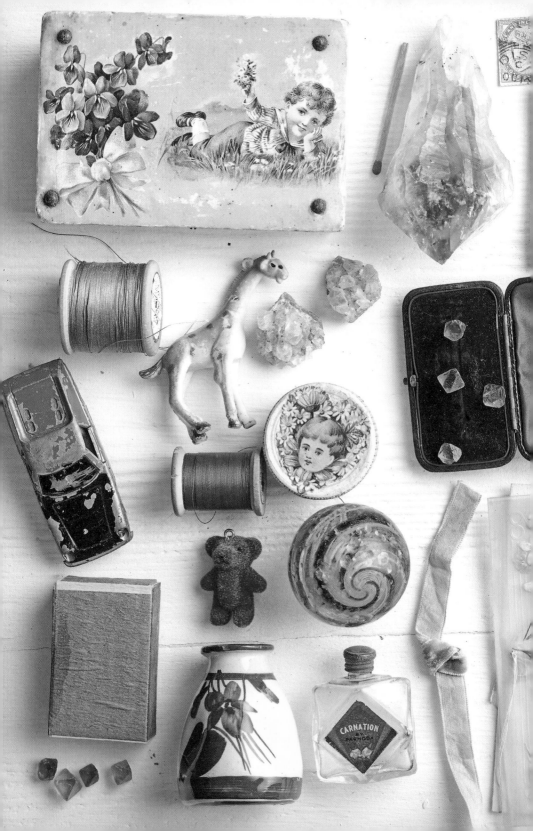

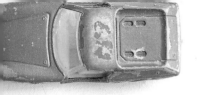

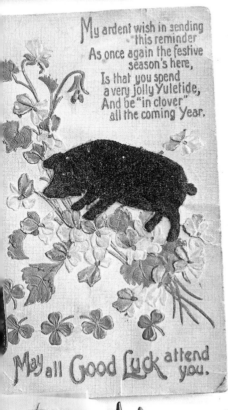

VIOLET

buddleia – mountain cornflowers –
globe artichokes – orchids – clematis
– pansies – violets – teasels – catmint
– violet sea snails – ochre sea stars –
wisteria – thistles – alliums – purple
starlings – plums – damsons – figs –
onions – irises – aubretias – lungwort
– lilacs – aubergines – red cabbages –
lavender – grapes – amethyst –
morning glory – dottyback fish –
magicians – ethereal – eccentric –
wizards – anemones – open-mindedness
– sweet dreams – wisdom – mystery
– insight – calmness – reflection

VIOLET

Violet is a colour of wisdom and mystery. Its hues
were often worn by royalty, priests and priestesses
and ceremonial magicians. When meditating, use
the colour to help you to be open and willing to
receive wisdom.

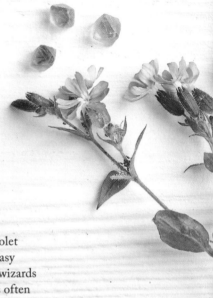

Seen as a magical colour with an ethereal quality, violet
shades are often used in art and film to portray fantasy
realms including fairy wonder worlds, dragons and wizards
adorned in violet cloaks. Wearing purple shades has often
been seen as slightly eccentric – another very good reason
to wear it.

On some social media sites in the USA, it was said that
painting your front door purple signified that 'a witch lives
here'. In some Pagan communities, purple ribbons are worn
to acknowledge Pagan Pride, worn at celebrations and
festivals. The colour was chosen as it suggests both open-
mindedness and spirituality.

The dreamlike quality of purple is often present for me
as I drift into sleep, like the hazy mauve hue that smoke
sometimes has. Jimi Hendrix was not wrong.

Try using the colour violet in some thoughtful, healing
incense meditation magic. Allow the wisdom or solution
you are asking for to gently flow into your mind, without
pressure, letting it float into your thoughts.

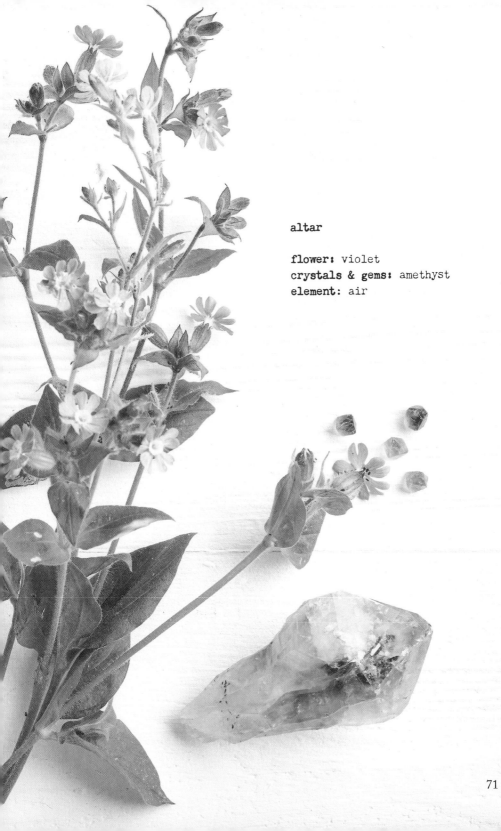

altar

flower: violet
crystals & gems: amethyst
element: air

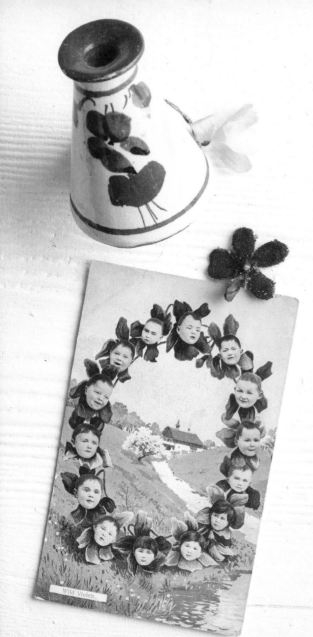

Wild Violets.

Violets

Violets, also known as sweet violets, have been in our lives forever. They are mentioned in Greek myth and in Shakespeare's plays. The Romans made violets into wine.

The scent of sweet violets is very strong, floral and woody and makes a perfect perfume. Many perfume houses across the world have a signature violet scent. Devon Violets brings back happy memories for me.

Violets have heart-shaped leaves, which are said to offer protection when dried, but the plant has many other beneficial attributes that can be called upon when making spells, charms and amulets.

Violets can be used to promote love, good luck, loyalty, modesty, faithfulness and the manifestation of wishes.

Placing violets under your pillow at night is said to encourage a restful night's sleep.

Violet Sleep Spell

Make a simple sachet from a thin cotton handkerchief or muslin to slip under your pillow at bedtime.

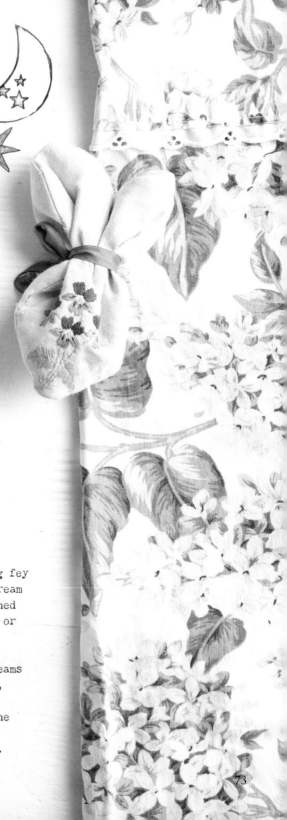

* 9 violet flowers and a few leaves
* clean tea towel
* 2 thin cotton handkerchiefs
* pins
* needle and thread

Gently wash the flowers and leaves, carefully patting them dry with a tea towel.

Place one of your handkerchiefs on your work surface, and put the flowers and leaves in the centre of the square.

Place the second handkerchief on top and pin the sides of the fabric together, making a sealed violet pouch.

Stitch in place and remove the pins.

Place the finished sachet under your pillow or next to where you sleep. Sweet dreams.

A Delicious Form of Night-time Magic

Dreams can slip away like the fleeting fey unless captured on paper, so keep a dream diary. Often our dreams are able to shed light on what we are feeling, needing or struggling with.

If the words don't come, draw your dreams instead... is there a symbol, a glyph, a face, a message? Make sure you date your dreams too. You could even use the notepaper on pages 156-157 to keep a record of your journeys through sleep.

Violet Sugar

Violet sugar is a sweet, fragrant treat that can add a little bit of extra magic to your baking. It can also be used to create a violet version of the Australian children's party staple known as Fairy Bread – simply sprinkle the sugar over buttered white bread for a delicious treat.

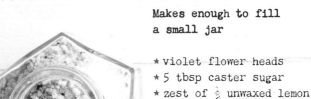

Makes enough to fill a small jar

* violet flower heads
* 5 tbsp caster sugar
* zest of $\frac{1}{2}$ unwaxed lemon

Rinse the flower heads and pat dry with a clean tea towel.

Add the violets, sugar and lemon zest to a deep bowl and blitz with a hand blender.

Sprinkle the mixture in a thin layer over a sheet of kitchen paper or a clean tea towel and leave to dry.

Sieve the sugar into a bowl.

Pour into a clean, sterilized jar and label.

Store in a cool, dry place and use within 2 weeks.

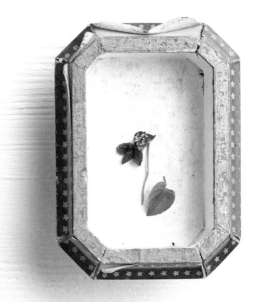

Candied Violets

The prettiest cake decorations.

* 1 egg white
* handful of violet flowers
* 1 tsp icing sugar

Whip the egg white in a shallow bowl until frothy.

Dip a flower into the whipped egg, tapping it on the side of the bowl to remove excess liquid, then transfer to a tray lined with baking paper.

Repeat with the remaining flowers and egg white.

Using a sieve, cloud your violets in icing sugar dust.

Leave them to dry on the tray for around 2 hours until crisp.

Store in a clean, sterilized jar and use within 2 weeks.

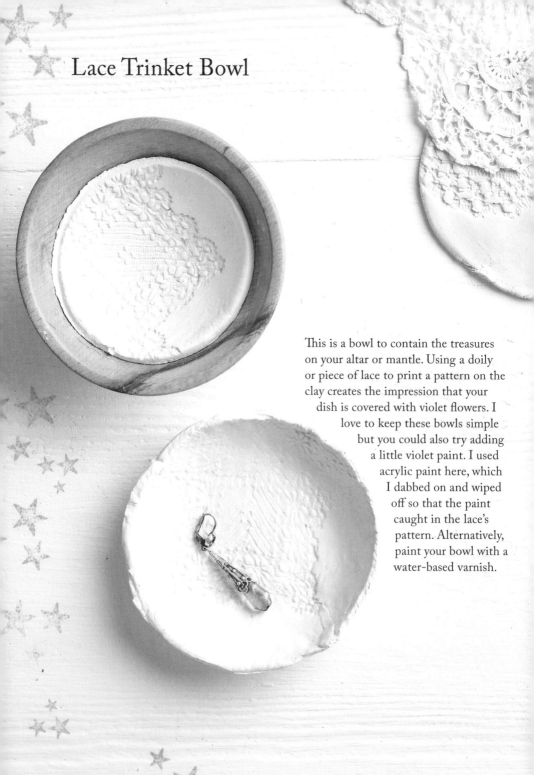

Lace Trinket Bowl

This is a bowl to contain the treasures on your altar or mantle. Using a doily or piece of lace to print a pattern on the clay creates the impression that your dish is covered with violet flowers. I love to keep these bowls simple but you could also try adding a little violet paint. I used acrylic paint here, which I dabbed on and wiped off so that the paint caught in the lace's pattern. Alternatively, paint your bowl with a water-based varnish.

* egg-sized piece of air-drying clay
* rolling pin
* doily or piece of old lace
* small bowl, about 7cm/2¾in in diameter
* knife

Take the clay and soften it between your hands, rolling it into a ball.

Roll out the clay until it is 5mm/¼in thick.

Place the doily or lace on your clay and run the rolling pin over the top, imprinting the pattern onto the clay.

Put your bowl over the clay, the bowl will act as a cutter to help you achieve a circular shape. Carefully cut around the rim using a knife.

Gently lay your clay circle inside your bowl so that the edges are raised.

Leave the clay in the bowl for a few days to dry.

Paint with a violet hue, if you like.

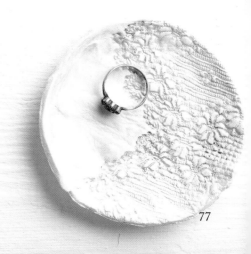

Violet Sigil

The shade is often thought of as a colour to help us concentrate on our third eye – which provides perception beyond ordinary sight – to uncover inner truths.

Violet and purple offer us wisdom and insight, healing and calm. Can this colour, its crystals and flowers and herbs aid you in your desires?

A simple sigil could be designed from a statement such as I AM WHOLE. You could also invest in some violet essential oil – just a drop can help you focus your mind and your senses.

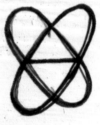

Decide on your intention.

Write it down.

I AM WHOLE

Remove the vowels and any repeated letters.

I̶ ̶A̶M̶ ̶W̶H̶O̶L̶E̶

Look at the letters you are left with.

M W H L

Draw your sigil on another piece of paper.

Try encircling your sigil in a circle to protect it. Making it whole.

Take a pencil, pen or pin, then scratch or draw your sigil onto a fresh violet candle.

Light with a match.

Breathe.

Concentrate on your inner wisdom.

Breathe.

Close your eyes.

Allow energy to fill you from the top of your head, gently encircling your body in violet light as you breathe in and out.

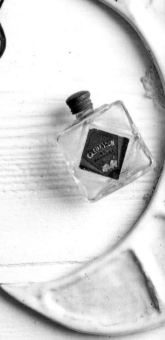

How are you feeling?
Make a note and mark the date.
If the words don't come, draw instead.

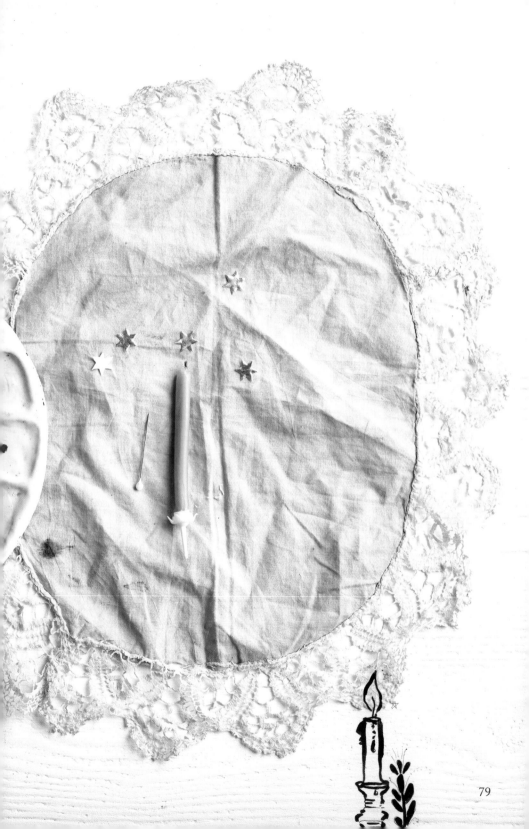

79

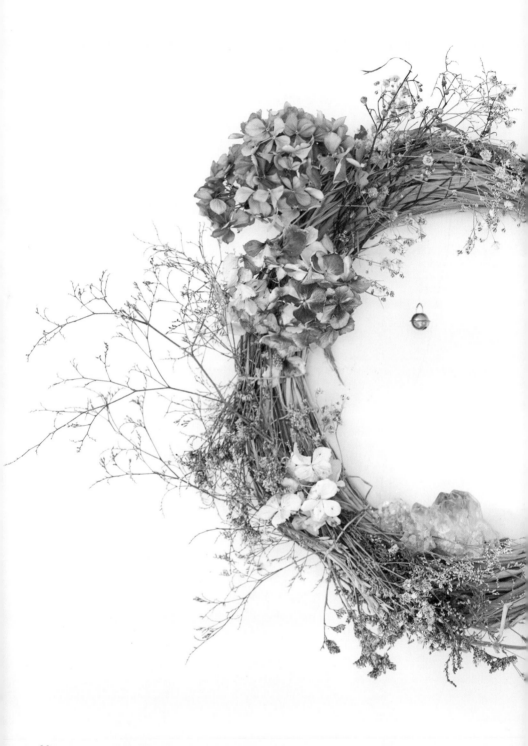

Amethyst Moon

Oh, how I love the moon. A crescent moon often symbolizes intuitiveness, fertility and the feminine. Amethysts are thought to have the power and wisdom to shield the wearer from negative energy. Often worn as an amulet, it is a stone associated with protection.

Here is a simple crescent moon make.

* 20 x 46-cm/18-in long willow sticks or lengths of straw
* wire
* scissors
* amethyst points and chips
* fresh or faux flowers and leaves
* bell or chime

Gather your sticks together and curve them into a crescent shape, securing them in place with wire and trimming away any excess willow or wire.

Once secured, decide which side will be the back, then thread a wire through the top. Make the wire long enough so you can hang your crescent on a wall or door.

Decorate your moon. Thread amethyst points, flowers and leaves through the willow and secure in place with wire.

If you are hanging your crescent on a door, add a bell or chime.

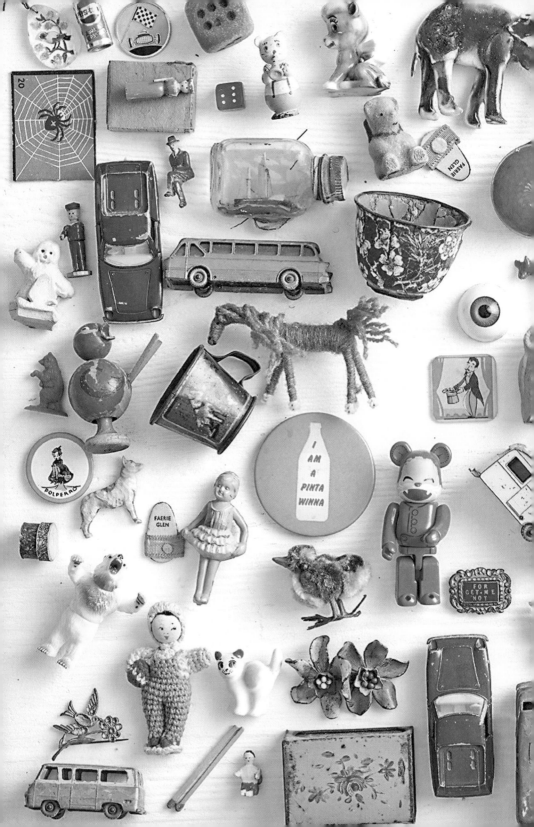

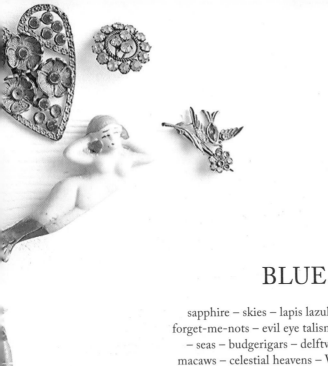

BLUE

sapphire – skies – lapis lazuli – bluebirds –
forget-me-nots – evil eye talisman – aquamarine
– seas – budgerigars – delftware – sapphire
macaws – celestial heavens – Willow pattern –
water – peacocks – Bristol glass – azure – cobalt
– sailor trousers – delphiniums – plumbago –
Himalayan blue poppies – indigo – bluebells
– ink – borage – peaceful – protection – blue
morpho butterflies – robin's eggs – turquoise
– lagoons – mermaids – royal blue – calming –
teal – cerulean – splendid fairy wrens – denim
– blue admiral butterflies – emergency lights
– blueberries – flames – hydrangeas – emperor
butterflies – blue crabs – blue jays – cornflowers
– kingfishers – midnight blue – tranquillity –
serenity – cooling – soothing – order – sadness
– reflection – healing – patience

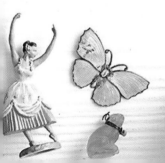

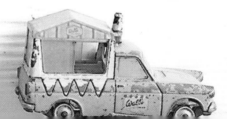

BLUE

Blue is a colour that can cool and calm an emotive situation and provide space for reflection. It's a colour of healing and patience ruled, of course, by water. In Victorian times, mourning rings were made from tiny turquoise stones in the shape of forget-me-not flowers, and allowed the wearer to keep a lost loved one in their thoughts.

Blue is often selected for its protective nature, it is the chosen colour of the universal evil eye talisman. It also lends a sense of responsibility and trust and features heavily in the uniforms of hospital staff.

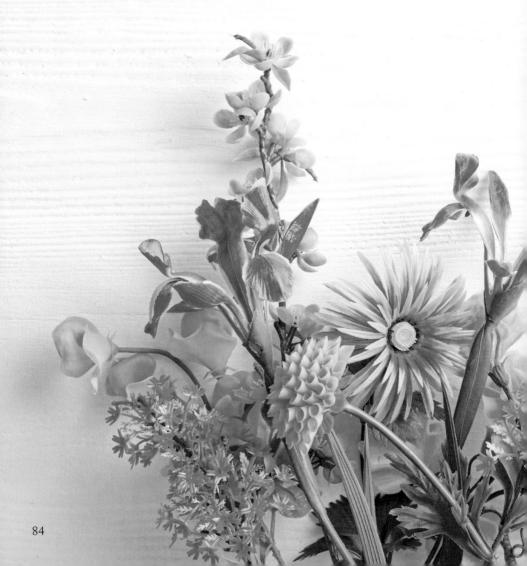

Artists are often drawn to its hues. Yves Klein stated that 'the Earth was entirely blue', and Joan Miró wrote that blue 'is the colour of my dreams' on a piece in 1925. And in medieval times, lapis lazuli was ground to a fine powder and used to paint the heavens in churches.

In nature, blue envelops us – we are surrounded by sea and sky. It brings to mind the realm of mermaids and lagoons, celestial stars, twilight and daydreaming. Using it in your spell work will help you to strengthen caring and creative intentions. It would appear that blue is our sky and the sky has no limit.

altar

flower: forget-me-not
crystals & gems: aquamarine, turquoise, sapphire
element: water

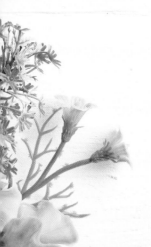

Stitch & Darn

I have always mended my favourite clothes. I've repaired and repaired them over and over I love them so much. I have a favourite needle, pins and my beloved scissors. When my mum died, I sat sewing for days and days, patching and darning an old holey frock that I love, using her black thread; sewing together the shock and grief as I tried to come to terms with her death. Grief is a spiteful beast. Sewing was a symbolic process for me then and continues to be so.

Stitching is a way I cast spells – each and every stitch has an intention. This page is about sewing together, closing a wound and attaching a kind or healing spell to an item of clothing or piece of fabric that means a lot to you. Louise Bourgeois's quote opposite says it all.

By embroidering a simple symbol, you can stitch a positive intention into your cloth:
♥ on a loved one's item of clothing to show affection - I embroidered a red heart, a little love spell, inside my partner's coat for a surprise Valentine's gift
☽ on the edges of bed pillows or pyjamas for sweet dreams
👁 embroidered on the end of your scarf to ward off negative energy

Forget-me-not Stitch

Forget-me-nots have long been used as a symbol of true love – a sign that a special person is always in your thoughts. Traditionally they have five petals, with a beautiful star and yellow eye in the centre. Use one to decorate your handkerchief or darn a hole.

* few strands of blue thread or silk

* 1 strand of yellow thread

* needle

Sew 5 petals in blue.

Add a stitch of yellow.

As you are stitching, think of loved ones passed, present and those who you will be meeting in your future.

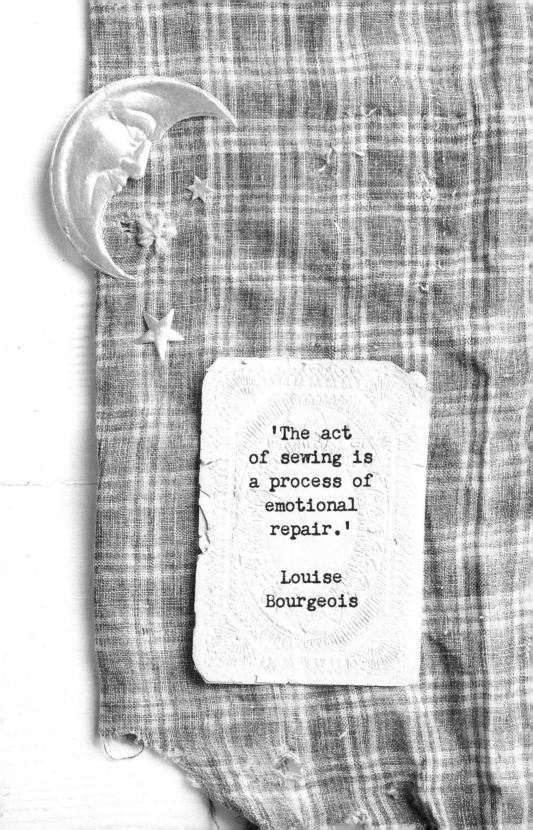

'The act
of sewing is
a process of
emotional
repair.'

Louise
Bourgeois

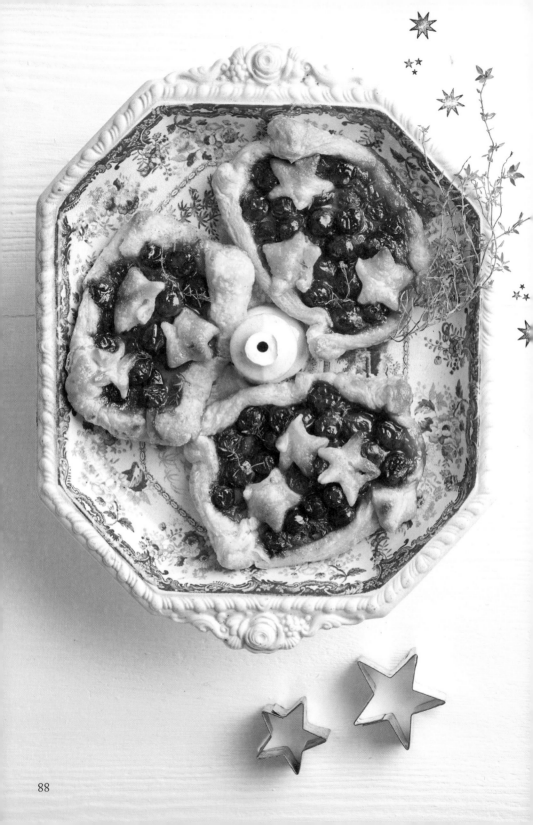

Star Tarts

Some situations call for something sweet and these delicious cosmic pastries cannot fail to bring comfort and joy.

* 200g/7oz blueberries
* 1 sprig of thyme, leaves removed
* 3 tbsp caster sugar
* 1 tbsp lemon juice
* pinch of salt
* 2 tbsp cornflour
* ¼ tsp ground cinnamon

* 1 large sheet of ready-rolled puff pastry (about 165g/5¾oz)
* 1 tsp butter
* 1 egg, lightly beaten
* icing sugar, for sprinkling
* clotted cream, to serve (see page 17)

Makes 4 tarts

Preheat the oven to 160°C/140°C fan/315°F/gas mark 2–3 and line two baking trays with baking paper.

Mix the blueberries, thyme leaves, caster sugar, lemon juice, salt, cornflour and cinnamon together in a bowl.

From the sheet of puff pastry, cut four rectangles, each one about 10 x 13cm/4 x 5in.

Using a small 1.5cm/⅝in biscuit cutter, cut out a few stars from the leftover pastry and leave them to one side.

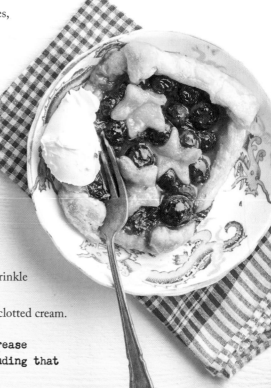

Divide the blueberry mixture evenly between the pastry rectangles, placing the mixture in the centre and leaving a pastry border of at least 2.5cm/1in around the sides.

Fold over the edges of the rectangles, by approximately 1cm/½in on all sides, to contain the mixture.

Dot with butter.

Pop a few pastry stars on top of each tart.

Brush the pastry with a little beaten egg and sprinkle with icing sugar.

Bake for 20 minutes or until golden. Serve with clotted cream.

Thyme is known as a herb that can increase communication into other worlds, including that of the kingdom of the fey.

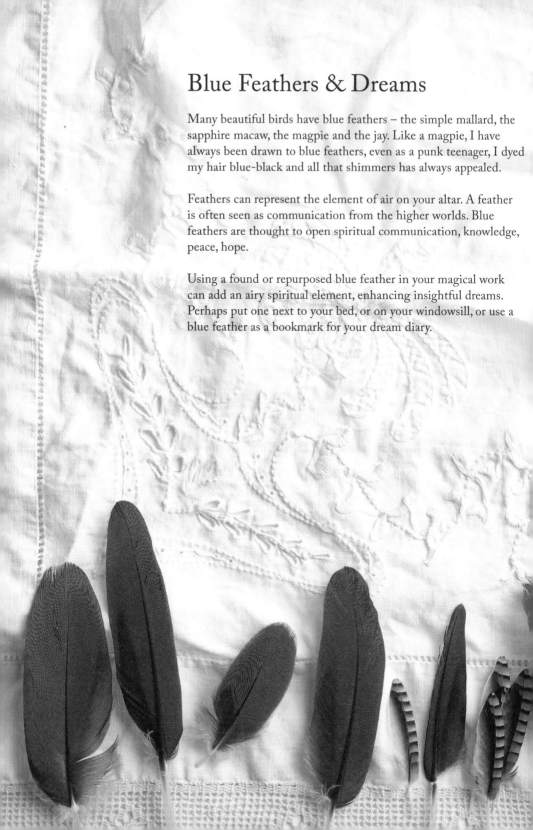

Blue Feathers & Dreams

Many beautiful birds have blue feathers – the simple mallard, the sapphire macaw, the magpie and the jay. Like a magpie, I have always been drawn to blue feathers, even as a punk teenager, I dyed my hair blue-black and all that shimmers has always appealed.

Feathers can represent the element of air on your altar. A feather is often seen as communication from the higher worlds. Blue feathers are thought to open spiritual communication, knowledge, peace, hope.

Using a found or repurposed blue feather in your magical work can add an airy spiritual element, enhancing insightful dreams. Perhaps put one next to your bed, or on your windowsill, or use a blue feather as a bookmark for your dream diary.

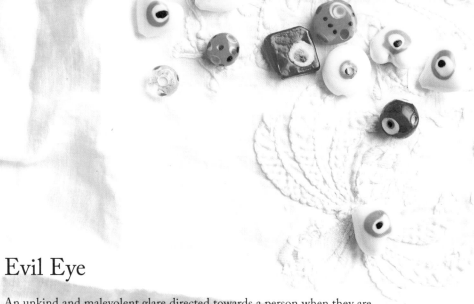

Evil Eye

An unkind and malevolent glare directed towards a person when they are unaware is known as the evil eye. I believe any ill-wisher to be unhappy or envious and sometimes there are ways you can tell if someone is casting the 'evil eye'. A heavy feeling or a large sigh within you can indicate the need to cleanse – that you are carrying someone else's emotional baggage. Jane Austen's brilliant quote from *Mansfield Park*, 'I was quiet but I was not blind', always reminds me of this.

These talismans or amulets depicting an eye, also known as 'evil eyes', are universal symbols of protection. The thinking is that they reflect the ill-wishers' negativity straight back at them in a glorious form of protective magic. **KAPOW!**

Very old talismans of the eye were created from clay, but glass evil eye beads were made popular and used by the Persians, Ottomans, Greeks and Romans. Blue glass evil eye beads can be found in every Mediterranean country but the symbol is also used worldwide. Try hanging one from a thread in your Crystal Grotto (see pages 60–61) or place upon your altar. Or tie evil eye beads on threads around your wrists, ankles and throat.

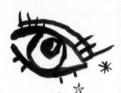

Eye Appliqué

Cut an eye shape in a plain fabric, then cut one
large circle and one small circle.

Stitch in place to create the iris and pupil.

Add some lashes - try using tiny bead sparkles to
decorate them.

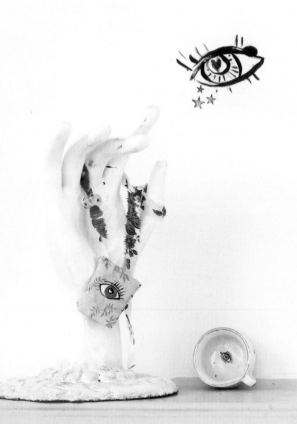

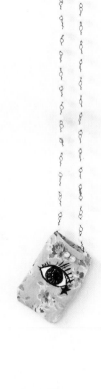

Spell Bag

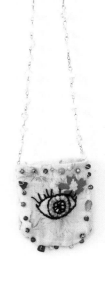

These bags are the perfect size to carry a crystal, talisman or charm but you can make the bag to any size. Larger bags are ideal for foraging twigs, sprigs, pebbles, herbs and treasure. Make it beautiful whatever size you decide upon.

* fabrics

* needle and thread

* pins

* length of string or braid (for the strap)

* acrylic paints and brush

* beads

Cut two pieces of fabric, each measuring 3 x 4cm/1¼ x 1½in.

Lay your two pieces of fabric right sides together.

Sew up three of the sides, leaving the shortest side at the top of the bag open.

Turn the bag inside out, and then fold in the top edges to create a hem, and pin in each end of your bag string. (You could even use an old necklace as a strap for your bag.)

Stitch firmly to secure the strap in place.

Embroider, paint or appliqué an eye symbol on one side.

Try stitching seed beads around your bag, attaching them in groups of three – with an odd one here and there – I'm a bit of a rebel.

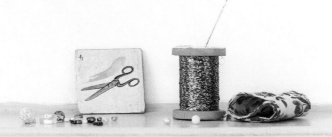

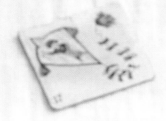

Blue Sigil

Blue as a colour, with its many tones, can help aid you in so many magical intentions. Blue can be soothing, calm, spiritual or refreshing. Are you flying high in the sky? Or leaping into a lagoon for a blast of freshness? Or peacefully, serenely floating?

Sometimes we are 'blue': down, low, depressed and sad. Remember you are cocooned and enveloped in blue by the sky. That the world is limitless. That there is change afoot. It will pass. I promise.

Let's try a gentle intention for our blue sigil example...
I AM SERENE

Remove the vowels and any repeated letters...
I̶ A̶M̶ S̶E̶R̶E̶N̶E̶

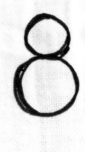

Look at the letters you are left with...
M S R N

Using these letters, design your sigil.
Use a pin on a fresh blue candle and scratch your sigil onto the side.
(Remember to make a note of this and date it.)
Sit quietly as you light your candle.
Allow yourself to relax from the top of your head to the tips of your toes.
Notice your breathing, in and out, nice and slowly.
Relax as you watch the flame, knowing all will be well.

When ready, extinguish the candle's flame.

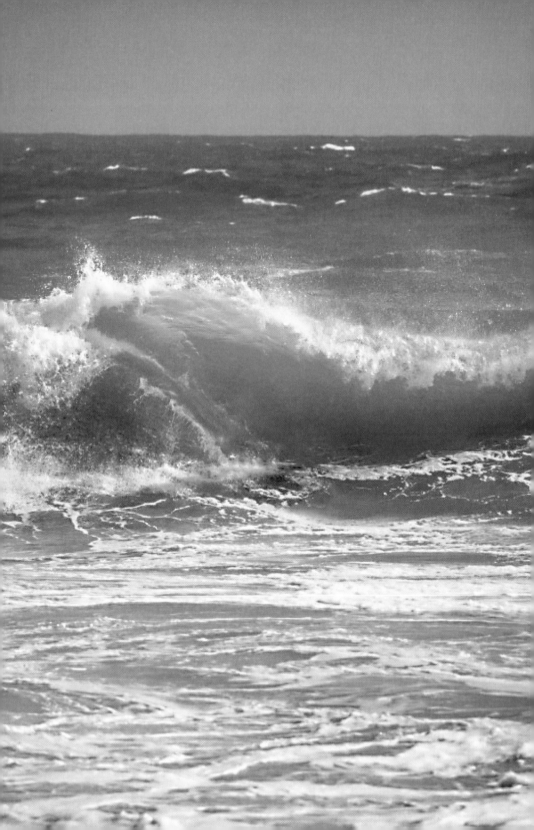

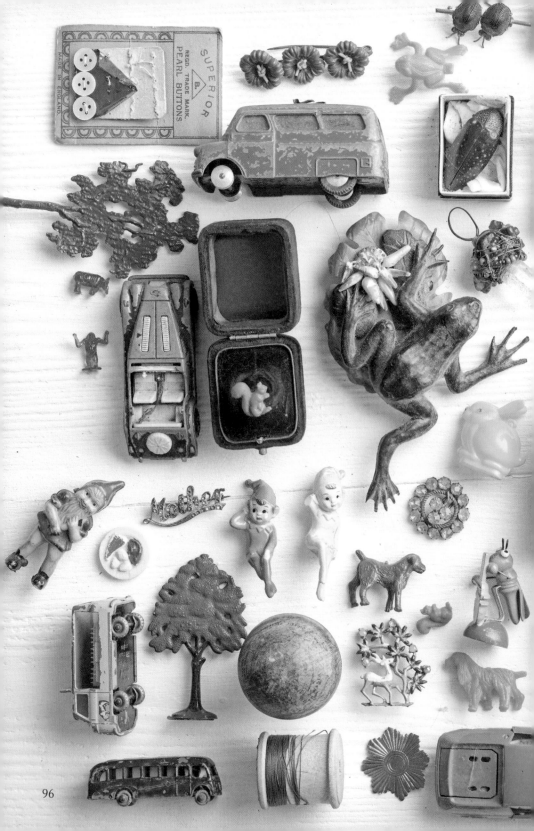

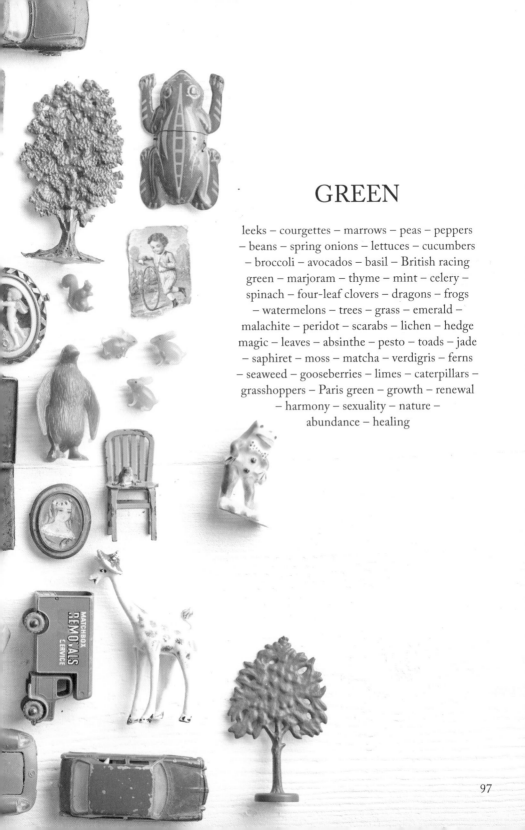

GREEN

leeks – courgettes – marrows – peas – peppers
– beans – spring onions – lettuces – cucumbers
– broccoli – avocados – basil – British racing
green – marjoram – thyme – mint – celery –
spinach – four-leaf clovers – dragons – frogs
– watermelons – trees – grass – emerald
malachite – peridot – scarabs – lichen – hedge
magic – leaves – absinthe – pesto – toads – jade
– saphiret – moss – matcha – verdigris – ferns
– seaweed – gooseberries – limes – caterpillars –
grasshoppers – Paris green – growth – renewal
– harmony – sexuality – nature –
abundance – healing

GREEN

Green is a colour of growth, sexuality, renewal, harmony and healing. Think curled new leaves, freshly cut grass, daisy-chain making and lying in meadows.

Green is also the colour of a strong natural magic that occurs in nature. Green magic or 'hedge magic' refers to the spells and healing charms cast by country-dwelling wise witches. Their skills are thought to have been passed down through their families for generations.

Often spells, charms, healing tinctures for animals and herbal medicines – drawing on the power of the moon, the tides and the sea – will be written or drawn into a family book, similar to a cookbook – as we know, so many recipes are also spells. Magic has been passed down to me from both sides of my family, through many generations. I treasure the book my mother gave to me.

Of course, not all hedge witches are countryside dwellers – there are plenty in towns and cities all over the world. Nature has a way of spreading through concrete and seeping through walls.

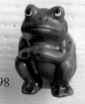

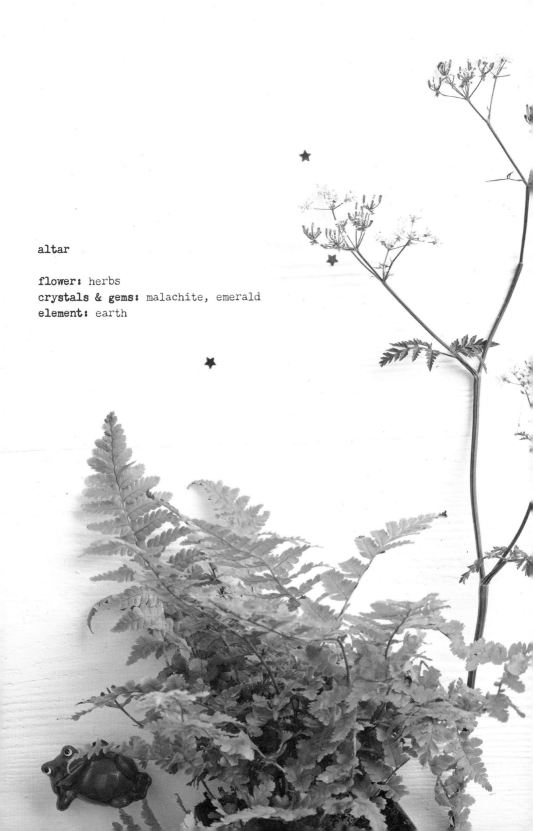

altar

flower: herbs
crystals & gems: malachite, emerald
element: earth

Language of Flowers

Meanings have been attributed to flowers for thousands of years. Here is my list to help you choose the right flowers for your altar and spell work.

ANEMONE	expectation
ANGELICA	inspiration
APPLE	magic, temptation
BASIL	strength, passion, energy
BAY	purification, spell holder
BERGAMOT	sleep, control issues
BLUEBELL	constant, reliable
BORAGE	stoic, standing ground
CAMOMILE	sleep, dreams, prophecy, calm
CARNATION	magical strength, mother, love
CEDAR	protection, invocation of spirits
CHRYSANTHEMUM	mourning, bravery, truth
CLEMATIS	thoughtfulness, beauty
CLOVER	animal blessings, protection of creatures, industry
DAFFODIL	regard, communication
DAISY	innocence, a reward
CYPRESS	money, healing
EUCALYPTUS	purification
FENNEL	sexuality, change, communication
FERN	sincerity
FORGET-ME-NOT	remembrance
GARDENIA	moon power
GERANIUM	laughter, happiness, movement
GOOSEBERRY	anticipation
HAWTHORN	hope, longing
HIBISCUS	delicacy, gentleness
HOLLYHOCK	feminine power, enchantment
HONEYSUCKLE	stability while changing
JASMINE	sexuality, dreams, love
JONQUIL	love's return
JUNIPER	strengthening of all magic, healing
LAVENDER	magic, clarity, calming, psychic dreams
LEMON	happiness, old magic and lore
LILAC	young love
LILY	sweetness
LILY OF THE VALLEY	happiness, weddings

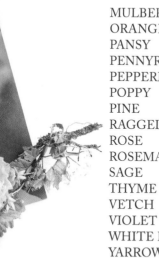

MULBERRY TREE	wisdom
ORANGE	energy, joy
PANSY	in my thoughts, friendship, affection
PENNYROYAL	reversal of negative energy, protection
PEPPERMINT	soothing, balancing
POPPY	plenty, courage, love
PINE	strength, youth
RAGGED ROBIN	wit and laughter
ROSE	attraction, fey, love, kindness, romance
ROSEMARY	memory, stimulation, energy, remembrance
SAGE	mental health, purification, cleansing
THYME	psychic ability, communications to other worlds
VETCH	thoughtfulness, shyness
VIOLET	love, innocence, magical, lore
WHITE HEATHER	luck, fairy flower
YARROW	wish granting, anger banishing
YEW	ancient profound wisdom, grief

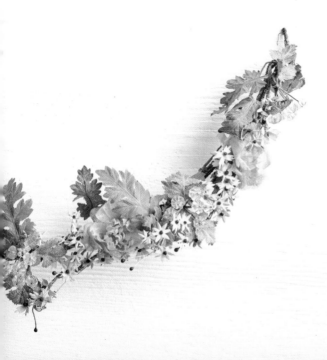

Green Bottle Candlestick

Fresh intentions. This candlestick can be used again and again for new spells.

Start by removing the label from the bottle. Soak the bottle in warm water and gently rub the label away (if a sticky residue is left behind, wipe the bottle with a little white spirit, then wash the bottle and your hands thoroughly).

Create a new label – you could draw, paint or print one.

Breathe.

Write a word on your label – this can be an intention or your focus whilst using your green candle.

I have used 'plenty' and 'new' here, as green can encourage abundance, but you could use any word such as 'fresh', 'renew' or 'growth'.

Secure your label to the bottle with glue. Surround it with paper flowers.

You could also use paper scraps, cut-outs, drawings and decorations, securing them in place with glue.

You could add a shell, securing it in place with glue.

You could also trail leaves and flowers around your bottle with some acrylic paint.

Once the bottle is decorated, trim the base of a green dinner candle so that it fits snugly and securely in the top of the bottle. I like to burn several different shades of green candles and let the wax drip down to create a 1970s bistro effect.

* old green bottle
* paper and pens
* paper flowers
* glue
* green dinner candle

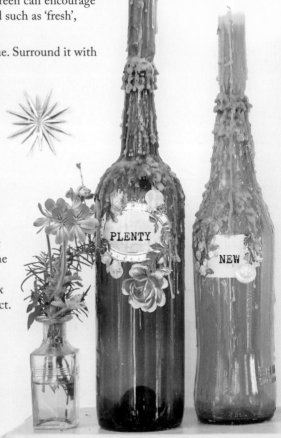

Candle Magic

Candle magic is such a simple but powerful way of casting a spell. The easiest way to explain candle magic is a birthday-cake wish – remember the importance of getting your wish just right, tightly closing your eyes, never revealing what you have wished for in case you jinx it and it doesn't come true? All of this passion and intensity is needed in candle magic. As we grow, we get the impression from society that wishing is for babies or just for birthdays, but a wish is a desire, an intention, a hope for change – and there is nothing babyish about change. Change takes courage. It is thoughtful and calm, but can also burn with desire.

Candle magic is driven by the element of fire but even an unlit candle can promote fine energy. I believe when casting any spell it's best to start afresh. A fresh candle signifies a fresh spell. (I buy short candles for this very reason.) Try always to use a fresh candle or at least cut the candle in half so you have a fresh wick. Old candles can carry energies from the last spell you used them for and may muddy your new intention. (Don't waste old candles, simply use them when you would like candlelight.) Whenever you perform candle magic, remember never to leave the flame untended. You should always be awake, aware and clear when performing candle magic.

* Find a quiet space.

* Visualize your intention or wish. What does it look like? What does it smell of? What colour is it?

* Choose a candle with a colour that supports your intention.

* Would you like to add a sigil to the candle to focus your intention further?

* Placing some crystals, herbs, flowers or charms near your candle can add extra power to your spell.

* Would you like to sprinkle some salt around yourself?

* Breathe.

* Light the candle and focus on your intention.

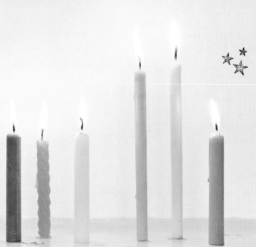

Herbs

For centuries, herbs have been used for cooking and for ritual and healing magic. You can make magical intentions when burning specific herbs. It can be a very energizing, thoughtful, inspiring and clarifying ritual. You'll need a fireproof bowl in a well-ventilated room.

Rosemary

Rosemary has often been thought to contain prophetic qualities and is also known as a plant of the fey – fairies are said to dwell beneath it. It is said that if you place a dish of flour under a rosemary plant on Midsummer's Eve, the following morning your true love's initials will be revealed.

I think of rosemary as the herb of remembrance, and for many centuries this herb has been associated with funerals and mourning. Sprigs were, and often still are, worn at funerals then thrown into the grave.

Bay Leaves

Bay, when burned, is a great anxiety lifter, helping to strip away unhelpful thoughts to clear your mind for future wishes.

Sigils can be drawn onto bay leaves before burning them: watch the release of smoke… send good wishes along with your intention to strengthen your desire and throw in a pinch of salt for some wisdom.

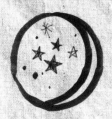

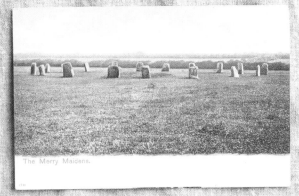

The Merry Maidens.

Sage

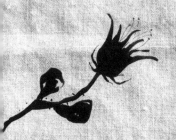

Sage has been used for centuries by Celtic Druids for rituals associated with cleansing, purification and repelling negative energy. This simple sage cleanse will clean your magical tools to remove the residue of past energies so you can start afresh with a new spell. Cleanse items such as scissors (used for cutting herbs, threads or paper sigils), crystals and wands.

Use some dried sage leaves and add a pinch of salt to boost this cleansing ritual.

* Breathe.
* Crush 6–8 sage leaves in the bowl.
* Light with a match.
* Throw in a pinch of salt if it feels right.
* Gently hold the items you wish to cleanse over the smoke.
* Visualize them being cleansed.
* Scoop some smoke with your hands over the crown of your head too.
* When you have finished, shake off the energy from your fingertips.
* Make sure the fire is completely out.

Wreath

This wreath is for life. You can use it as you would an altar and decorate it seasonally – using fresh leaves, herbs, flowers, crystals, stars, magical symbols and hag stones. I like to add paper fortunes from fortune cookies and old valentine cards, too.

* metal coat hanger
* 26cm/10½in willow wreath
* pliers and scissors
* wire
* moss
* faux flowers and leaves
* small treasures – such as old Christmas decorations, toys, fripperies, dried flowers
* paper decorations – such as flowers, butterflies
* pins with coloured heads
* glue gun and glue sticks

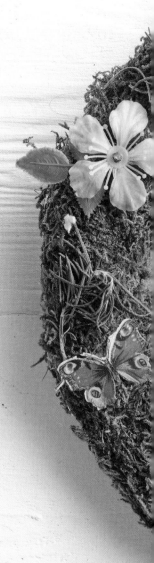

Bend your coat hanger into a circle with the hook at the top (use pliers if you need to).

Fasten the wreath to the coat hanger by winding wire around the wreath and the hanger, making sure the hook is at the top of the wreath.

Cover your wreath with moss.

Once secure, you can decorate the wreath, using the glue gun and glue sticks, pins and wire to secure your decorations in place.

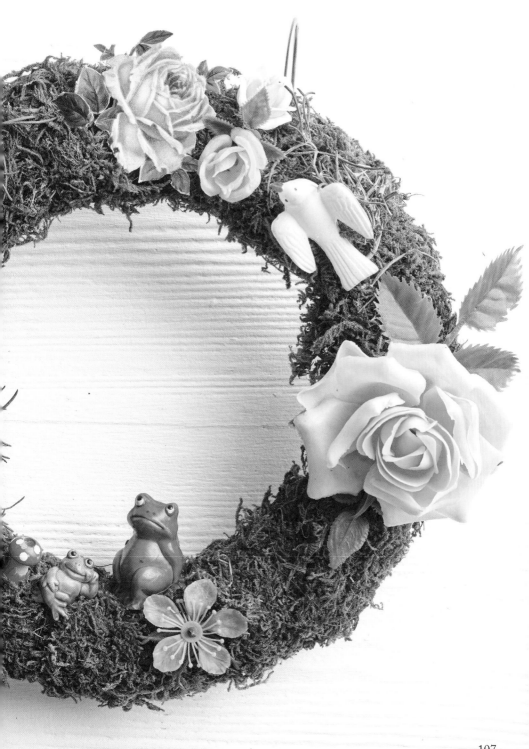

Mint Tea

For many centuries, mint has been known as a soothing and purifying herb. As well as smelling wonderful it is magnificent for nausea and digestion. Uplifting and refreshing, it's perfect added to herb salsa, pickled in vinegar as a sauce, or chopped into a pan of buttered potatoes. And, of course, it makes delicious tea – a complete sensory herbal tonic.

* bunch of fresh mint
* juice of ½ lemon
* sugar

Fill a tea glass with fresh mint.

Add boiling water and steep for a few minutes.

Add a squeeze of lemon juice and sweeten to taste with sugar.

Mint is also a very satisfyingly easy herb to grow, flourishing and spreading even in small pots on windowsills. Add a few sprigs to a tepid bath on a hot night – it's remarkably cooling.

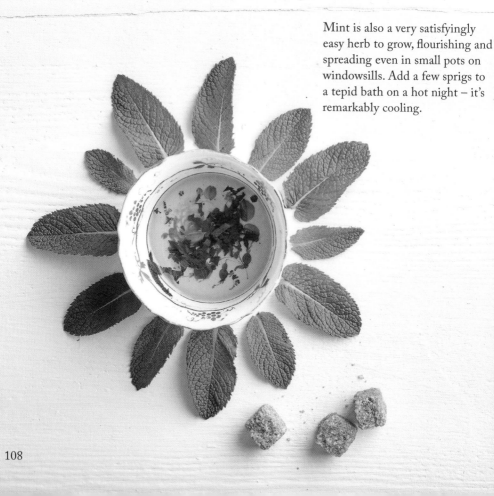

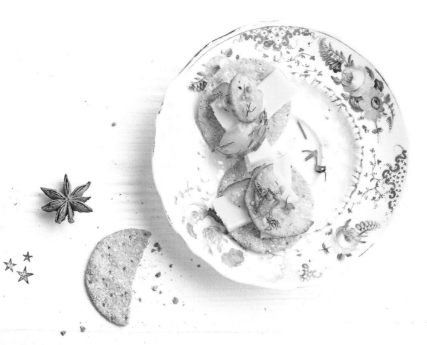

Cucumber Pickle

This pickle is completely delicious on top of salads, with yogurt as an alternative to tzatziki, and with cheese and crackers.

Makes enough to fill a large jar

* ★ 3 cucumbers
* ★ salt
* ★ 1 shallot, peeled and finely chopped
* ★ 2 tsp mustard seeds
* ★ 2 star anise
* ★ 3 sprigs of fresh dill
* ★ ½ tsp white pepper
* ★ ½ tsp turmeric
* ★ 5 tbsp caster sugar
* ★ 150ml/5¼fl oz/scant ⅔ cup vinegar

Slice the cucumbers thinly and sprinkle with salt.

After 40 minutes, rinse thoroughly and pat dry.

Combine all the ingredients in a saucepan and bring to the boil, then remove from the heat and leave to cool.

Transfer to a large, sterilized jar and secure the lid tightly.

Store in the fridge and use within 1 month.

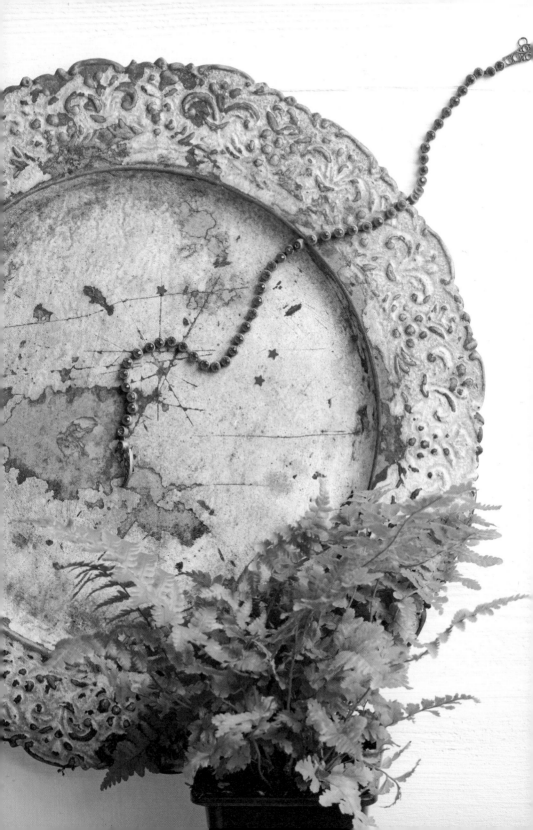

Green Sigil

What kind of intention would you like to make?
Walk outside into nature and using the colour green
that represents fresh new starts and vibrant, ripe
energy, decide upon your intention or wish.

Decide on your intention.

Write it down...
I AM HAPPY

Remove the vowels and repeated letters...
~~I AM HAPPY~~

Look at the letters you are left with...
M H P Y

Work these letters into a sigil – try adding plant-
like fronds or leaves to your design.

Breathe.

Try drawing your sigil onto a living leaf – gardens,
parks, hedges and the countryside are all great. As
your leaf continues to grow, your sigil will too.

Remember your sigil may change. What seemed
perfect and forever yesterday may not be relevant
today and that's fine... you can create as many
as you like.

You could also use a green stone or gem
to activate your sigil. Draw on your
symbol – as it fades your sigil will
be released. Malachite is one of my
favourites, known to open the wearer to
love, loyalty and trust.

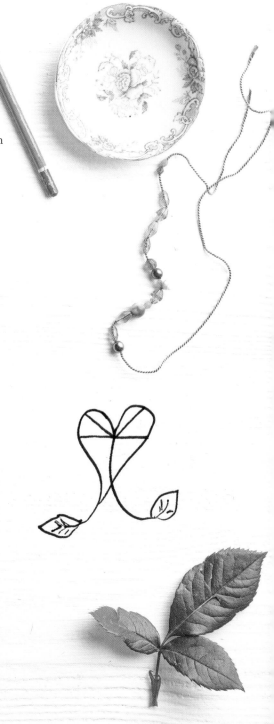

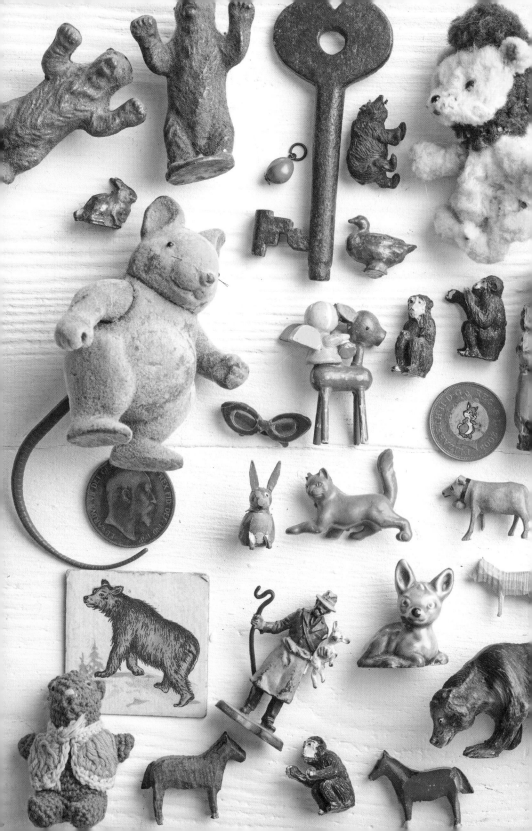

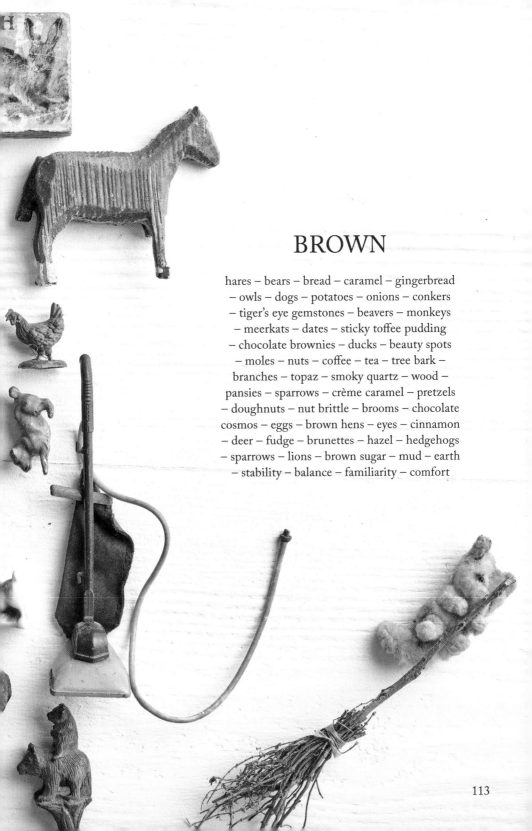

BROWN

hares – bears – bread – caramel – gingerbread
– owls – dogs – potatoes – onions – conkers
– tiger's eye gemstones – beavers – monkeys
– meerkats – dates – sticky toffee pudding
– chocolate brownies – ducks – beauty spots
– moles – nuts – coffee – tea – tree bark –
branches – topaz – smoky quartz – wood –
pansies – sparrows – crème caramel – pretzels
– doughnuts – nut brittle – brooms – chocolate
cosmos – eggs – brown hens – eyes – cinnamon
– deer – fudge – brunettes – hazel – hedgehogs
– sparrows – lions – brown sugar – mud – earth
– stability – balance – familiarity – comfort

BROWN

Brown is the colour of the earth, the ground beneath our feet, the strong tree trunks and gentle animals. It is a colour of profound stability, familiarity and comfort. It's very stabilizing and 'grounding' for the soul.

The colour brown reminds me of joyous childhood memories of making mud pies, and today I still immerse my hands in the earth as I plant my herbs and flowers.

Pansies, one of my favourite flowers, often appear in shades of brown. 'Pansy' derives from the French *penser*, which means 'to think about or ponder'. They were often given by suitors as a symbol that they were thinking of the recipient.

altar

flower: pansy
crystals & gems: tiger's eye gemstone
element: earth

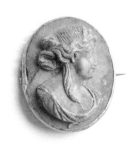

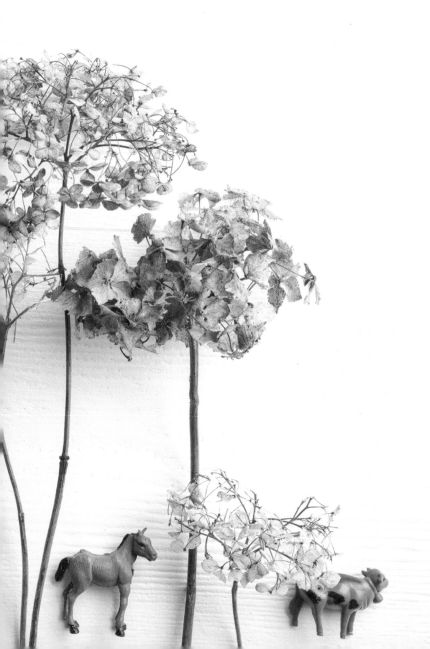

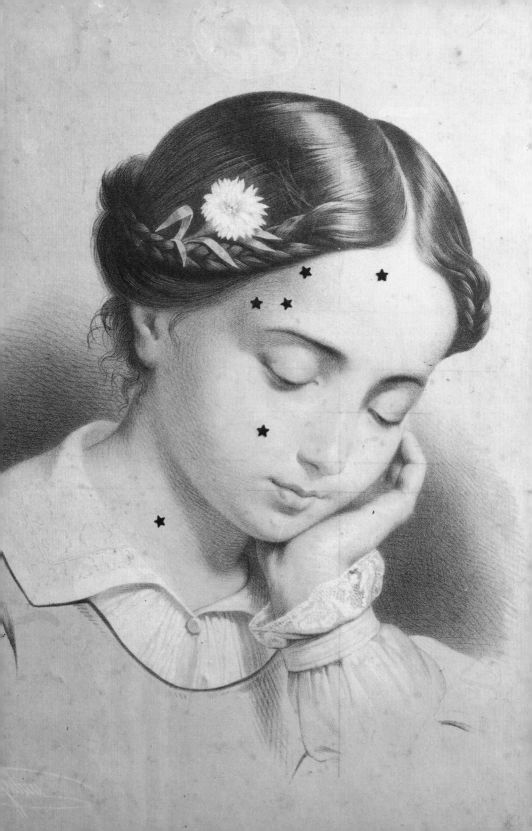

Beauty Spots

As a woman with plenty of moles – and two prominent ones on my face – I have always been a little defensive about them. When I was little, when other children were cruel and called me 'warty' or 'witch', my family taught me to reply promptly, 'I have beauty spots'. As a teenager I would darken them with my eyeliner and rather adored them. They have become more pronounced over the years and at one point I considered having them removed – not because they posed a health risk but because I felt pressured to meet society's beauty standards and have smooth, flawless skin. As I reach 56, I find I rather love them. They are such an intrinsic part of my essence and I now wear them with pride.

For many centuries, beauty spot patches were applied to cover pockmarks or to make the wearer seem more beautiful. Ancient Romans wore patches made from leather to cover scars, and Hippocrates had a theory that mole placement was linked to the planets in astrology. In Chinese fortune-telling the particular position of a mole is thought to signify certain fortunes.

In the eighteenth century, fake beauty spots (or mouches) – made from clippings of black velvet, silk, satin and even mouse skin – were in fashion. The position of a beauty spot was thought to convey a coded message, such as which political party you aligned yourself with and affairs of the heart. A magazine from 1787 suggested nine positions for the spots that, if used, would protect a woman from earning a scurrilous reputation.

Corner of eyelid	passionate
Centre of forehead	majestic
Dimple formed by smile	happy
Middle of cheek	gallant
Corner of mouth	kiss
Near nose	brisk
On lip	coquettish
Under lip	discreet
On pimple	concealing

In medieval Europe, malevolent witch finders called moles 'witches' teats' and thought that imps and familiars fed from them. A mole was regarded as proof that a woman was a witch and we know from history what horrors happened next.

Brown Sigil

Brown is the colour of the earth and so it will help to strengthen intentions focused on stability and balance. Why not try activating your sigil by drawing it on a pot you're planting up? This will provide positive energy for yourself and for the seeds or plant you are growing. Remember to nurture your plant and yourself. You could also draw your sigil directly into the earth, on a path in chalk, or on a plant marker.

Breathe.

Decide on your intention or wish, for example...

I AM GROUNDED

Write your intention down on paper.

Remove the vowels and any repeated letters...

~~I AM GROUNDED~~

Look at the letters you are left with and create your sigil...

M G R N D

Breathe.

Activate your sigil and allow yourself to grow.

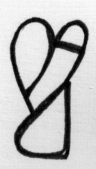

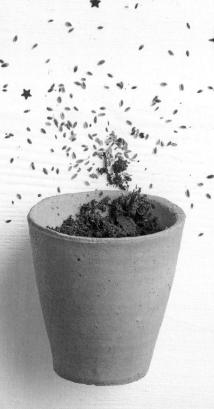

Hazelnut Brittle

This is a great gift and the perfect snack to take to a firework display or on a picnic. The brittle is also delicious served with coffee or sprinkled on top of cakes. Any nuts will work.

Makes 8–10 servings

* 200g/7oz hazelnuts
* 200g/7oz/1 heaped cup caster sugar (muscovado or soft brown sugar works well too)

Preheat the oven to 160°C/140°C fan/315°F/gas mark 2–3 and line two trays with baking paper.

Spread the nuts over one of the lined trays and bake for 8–10 minutes.

Tip the hot hazelnuts into a clean tea towel and vigorously rub them – this will remove some of the skins, but don't worry about removing the skins entirely.

Pour the hazelnuts and sugar into a saucepan. Cook over a medium-high heat, stirring continuously with a wooden spoon. After a while the sugar will begin to caramelize.

Continue to stir until the sugar has melted.

Once you have a pan of caramel-coated nuts, pour them onto the second lined tray to cool.

Once cool, chop roughly and store in an airtight container for up to 2 weeks.

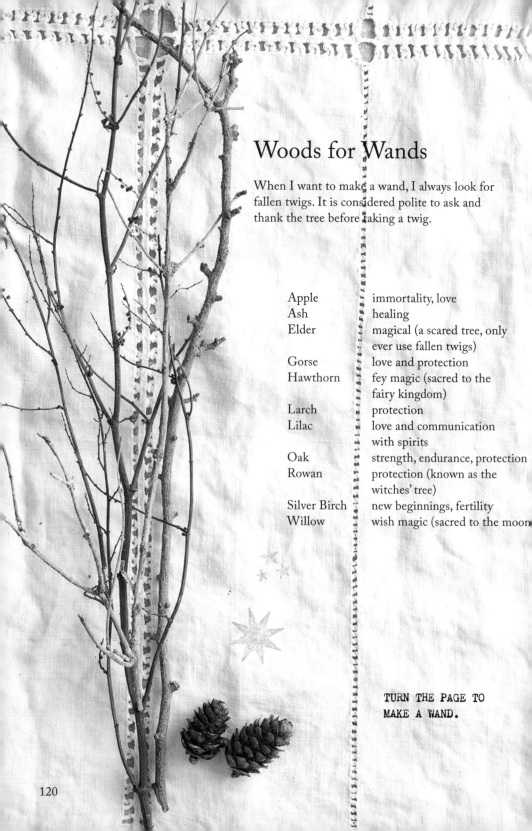

Woods for Wands

When I want to make a wand, I always look for fallen twigs. It is considered polite to ask and thank the tree before taking a twig.

Apple	immortality, love
Ash	healing
Elder	magical (a scared tree, only ever use fallen twigs)
Gorse	love and protection
Hawthorn	fey magic (sacred to the fairy kingdom)
Larch	protection
Lilac	love and communication with spirits
Oak	strength, endurance, protection
Rowan	protection (known as the witches' tree)
Silver Birch	new beginnings, fertility
Willow	wish magic (sacred to the moon

TURN THE PAGE TO MAKE A WAND.

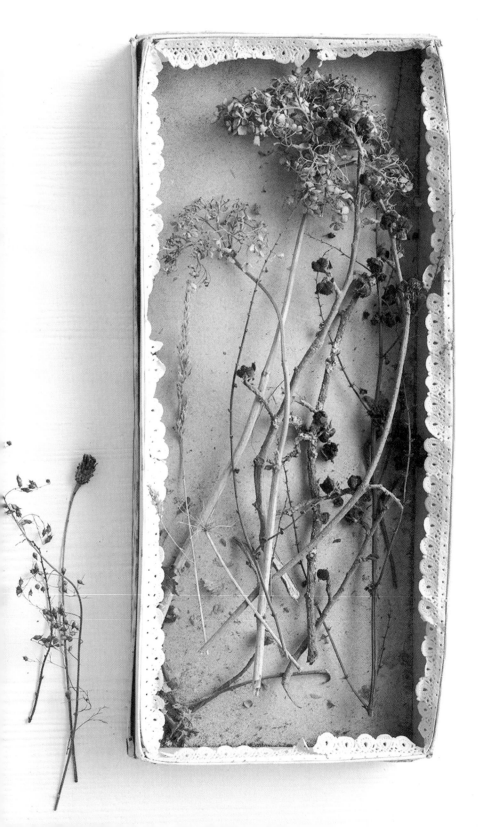

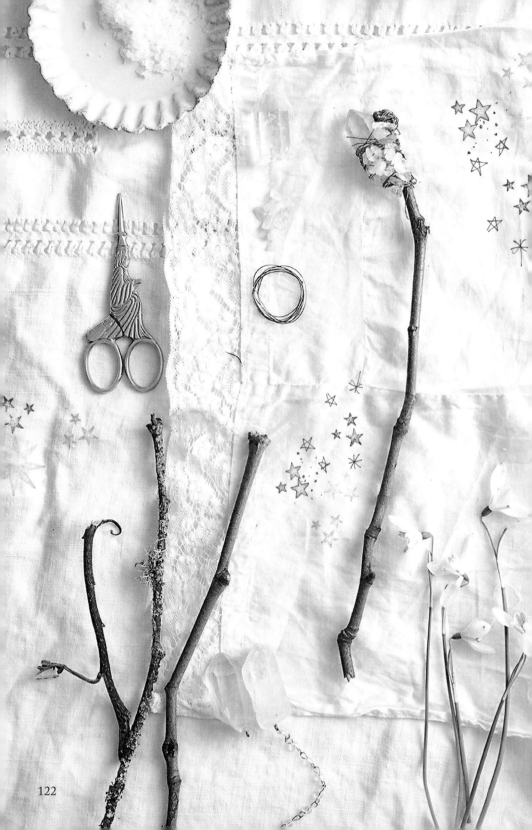

Making a Wand

A wand can help direct your intention using the power of colour, wood and crystal. Here's how to make one.

* rock crystal point with a hook (crystals sold as keyrings often have one)
* fallen twig
* 26 or 28 gauge wire, any metal (copper is my favourite)
* scissors
* small crystal beads, optional

Cut a 50cm/20in piece of wire.

Bend it in half and then thread one end through the hook of the crystal so the crystal sits in the centre of the wire. (You should have two lengths of wire either side of the crystal.)

Firmly wrap the right-hand wire around the crystal to secure it to the twig tip while holding the crystal firmly in place with your other hand.

Continue to wrap until the crystal is secured at the desired angle. If your crystal feels wobbly or loose, wrap more wire around it. Try not to succumb to glue!

Add a few extra crystal beads, if you fancy, and secure in place with wire.

If it feels right, you could add a few seasonal flowers, grasses or faux flowers to your wand.

Cleansing your crystal before you begin making your wand is a good idea. To cleanse with running water, hold your crystal under the cold tap and leave it to dry in sunlight or moonlight to recharge. Alternatively, cleanse your crystal with a sea salt wash - put a pinch of sea salt in a bowl of water and wash your crystal before leaving it to dry and recharge as above.

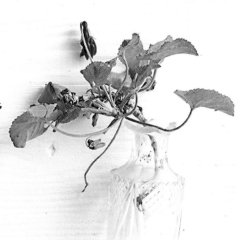

Sacred Trees

Trees are important symbols of life, death and rebirth. Shamanistic rituals often use trees as a ladder or portal to descend or ascend to different worlds, to greet animal spirits, the fey, or ancient ancestors. Imagine trees as a lift or staircase to three floors: the lower floor is often where you will meet your animal spirit; the middle floor is our daily reality; and the upper is where we meet with higher energies, angels and sometimes ourselves.

One of the most famous trees is Yggdrasil - a mythical Norse tree so powerful that it linked the heavens, the gods, the underworld and the world of humans. Thought by some to be a great ash, most believe it was actually a vast yew.

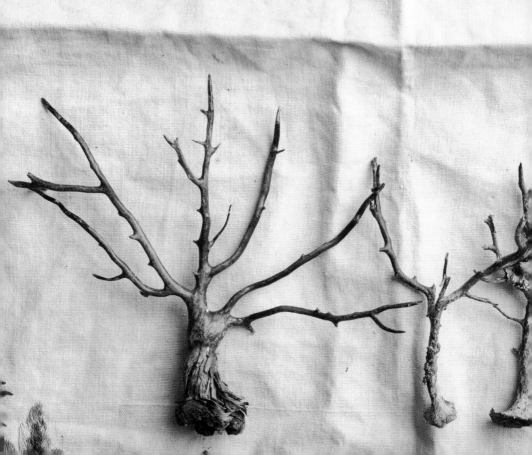

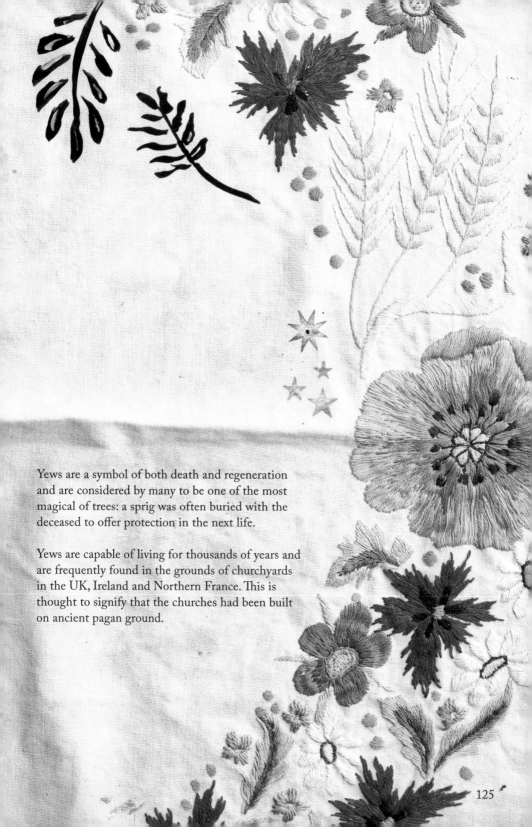

Yews are a symbol of both death and regeneration and are considered by many to be one of the most magical of trees: a sprig was often buried with the deceased to offer protection in the next life.

Yews are capable of living for thousands of years and are frequently found in the grounds of churchyards in the UK, Ireland and Northern France. This is thought to signify that the churches had been built on ancient pagan ground.

125

Animal Spirit Guides

For centuries, Shamans worldwide have practised the art of journeying to meet their animal spirit guides. You should use a qualified practitioner to make the journey to meet your spirit animal (see page 158). Often this journey begins with the practitioner drumming to lead you into a meditative state – a gentle trance that takes you into a different world where you can meet your guide.

Meeting your animal spirit guide can be quite a surprise. You may have an idea that your animal will be an X or a Y, as I did, but when you finally meet them there is an 'Ah, of course' moment. Suddenly you will see this particular creature everywhere and it will provide an incredible sense of comfort and belonging. It is a very personal bond and I was advised not to tell others the nature of my animal, but instead keep its identity close to my heart. You can call on your spirit animal, politely, when you need help with a problem or reassurance. I have received abundance when needed from mine. Always thank them.

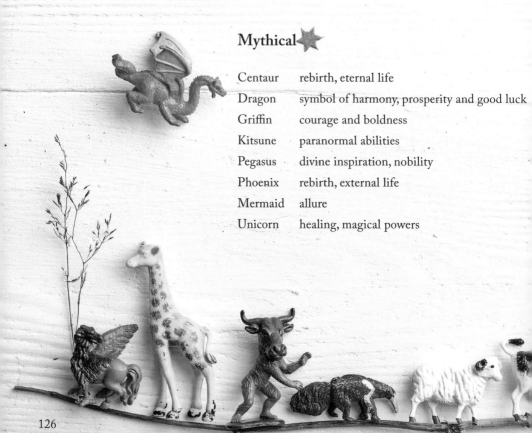

Mythical

Centaur	rebirth, eternal life
Dragon	symbol of harmony, prosperity and good luck
Griffin	courage and boldness
Kitsune	paranormal abilities
Pegasus	divine inspiration, nobility
Phoenix	rebirth, external life
Mermaid	allure
Unicorn	healing, magical powers

Animal

Badger   practitioner in the knowledge of herb magic and lore
Bat   guardian of the night
Bear   strength, spiritual journeying
Butterfly transformation
Cat   wisdom, knowledge of inner self, balance
Cow   tradition, patience
Crow   keeper of the knowledge of sacred lore
Deer   animal guide of the goddess of the moon
Dog   loyalty
Duck   spirit of those passed on
Fish   ability to hide emotional pain
Frog   abundance, foreteller of rain
Hare   fertility
Horse   healing, enlightenment
Lizard   conversation
Mouse   scrutiny, detailed thinking
Otter   curiosity
Owl   able to see what others can't, wisdom
Pheasant confidence
Rabbit   protection during childbirth
Snake   life, death, rebirth
Tiger   fierce, strong, courage, release of fear
Wolf   teacher

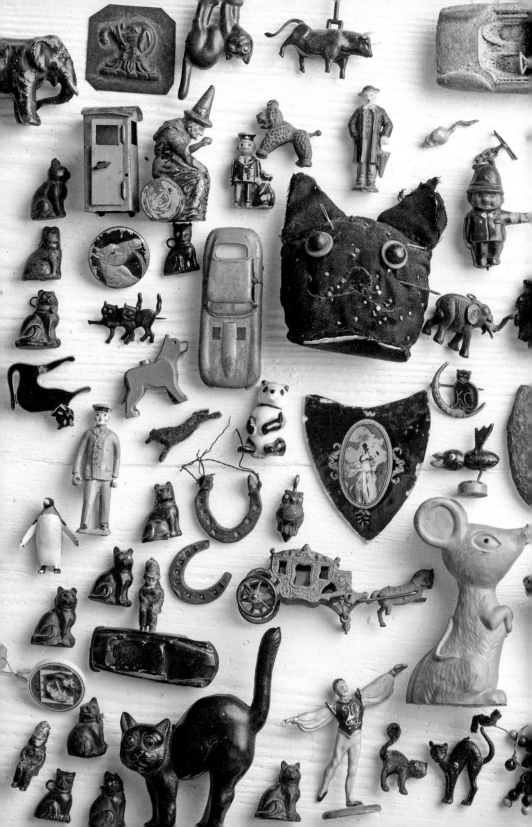

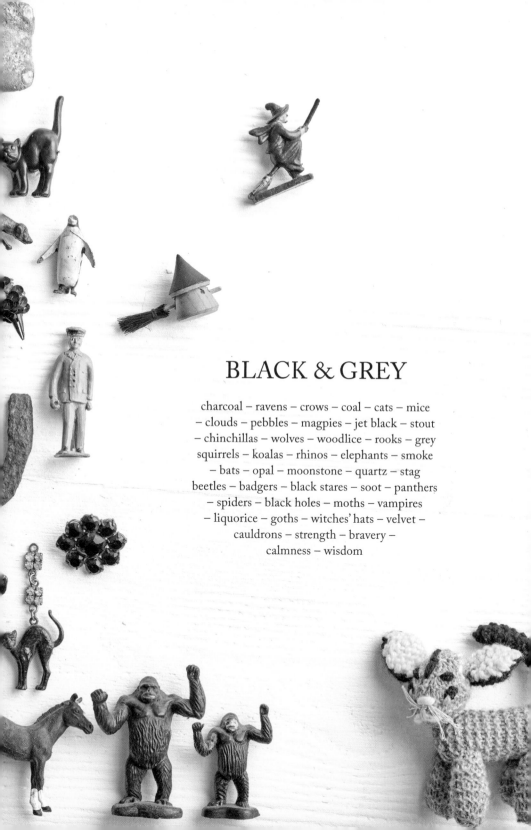

BLACK & GREY

charcoal – ravens – crows – coal – cats – mice
– clouds – pebbles – magpies – jet black – stout
– chinchillas – wolves – woodlice – rooks – grey
squirrels – koalas – rhinos – elephants – smoke
– bats – opal – moonstone – quartz – stag
beetles – badgers – black stares – soot – panthers
– spiders – black holes – moths – vampires
– liquorice – goths – witches' hats – velvet –
cauldrons – strength – bravery –
calmness – wisdom

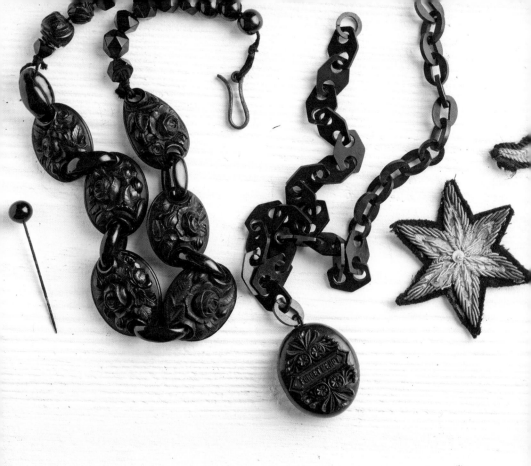

BLACK & GREY

Historically, black and grey have been associated
with the idea of 'black magic' – a practice thought
to conjure evil spirits for self-serving purposes.
However, when used kindly, black and grey can help
us to feel stronger, braver and calmer. I find both
colours grounding and a good base for magical work.

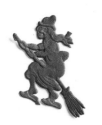

Though black can be the colour of secrecy, it also has authority and will help you to stand tall and hold your ground. It also has a sophisticated, sexy, but soothing nature too. Grey has softer qualities and can balance and cool our thoughts. Grey is a traditionally calming colour, often used in our homes; it is said to have beneficial restorative power. It's also a colour of compromise and control and can help us to receive insightful advice.

Black and grey are very good colours for intentions made to ward off negativity, summon courage and seek clarity.

altar

flower: 'Queen of Night' tulip
crystals & gems: moonstone
element: fire

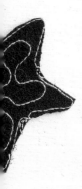

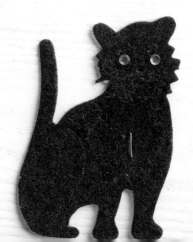

131

Stout Cake

A grown-up cake with a hint of chocolate. Unusual and moreish, it adds a little drama to the tea table.

Serves 10

For the cake
* 250ml/8¾fl oz/generous 1 cup Irish stout
* 250g/9oz salted butter, plus extra for greasing
* 160ml/5½fl oz/⅔ cup sour cream
* 2 eggs, lightly beaten
* 80g/2¾oz/heaped ¾ cup cocoa powder
* 390g/13¾oz/scant 2¼ cups caster sugar
* 280g/10oz/heaped 2 cups self-raising flour

For the icing
* 140g/5oz/1 cup icing sugar, sifted
* 280g/10oz/1¼ cups cream cheese
* 1 tsp cornflour
* 110ml/3¾fl oz/½ cup whipping cream

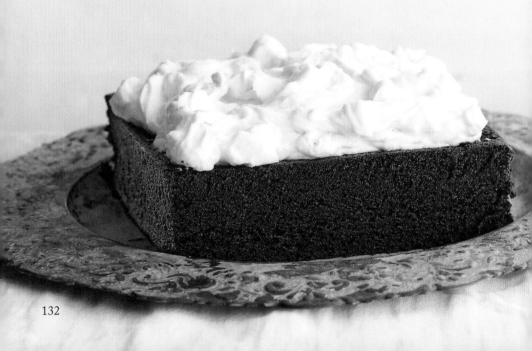

Preheat the oven to 160°C/140°C fan/315°F/gas mark 2–3.

Grease and line a 23-cm/9-in cake tin.

Pour the stout into a saucepan and add the butter. Warm over a low heat, stirring gently until the butter has melted.

Mix the sour cream and eggs in a large bowl, then add the cocoa and sugar and stir until combined.

Pour the stout and butter mixture into your bowl and whisk until smooth. Fold in the flour.

Pour the mixture into your prepared tin.

Bake for 50 minutes to an hour until a skewer inserted into the centre of the cake comes out clean. Remove from the oven and leave to cool in the tin.

While the cake cools, make the icing. Whisk the icing sugar, cream cheese and cornflour together in a bowl.

In another bowl, whisk the whipping cream until you have soft peaks, then fold both mixtures together.

Liberally ice the top of your cooled cake.

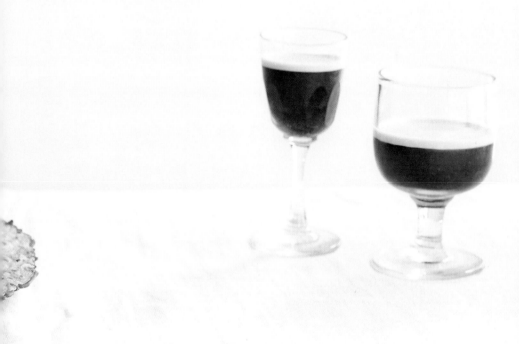

Runes

Runes are not for fortune-telling. Instead, the stones awaken your own intuition and the reading of runes requires quiet concentration. Runes are a good way of focusing on any questions you may have or for searching for future possible outcomes. Runes are a great way of grounding you, helping you pause from your busy life by pulling you back down to earth and allowing you to rest for a moment. I often ask the runes for insight on how I am faring rather than a specific query.

Each rune bears a magical symbol, possessing its own unique power. Making your own set of runes will give you a more accurate reading, as they are fully in tune with your own intentions. I favour creating runes using natural pebbles and stones, but you could also make them from clay or wood. I use a fibre-tip pen to draw on my symbols. Keep your runes in a small bag, wrapped in a white cloth that can also be used to cast them upon.

Here are the symbols – and their meanings – that you should include in your set to help you interpret the answer to your questions:

ᚠ	FEOH	nourishment, reward, wealth, fed
ᚢ	UR	virility, fertility
ᚦ	THORN	temptation, warning
ᚩ	OS	spoken wisdom, a message
ᚱ	RAD	union or reunion
ᚲ	KEN	enlightenment
ᚷ	GYFU	love, forgiveness, a gift
ᚹ	WYN	sate, love, light
ᚻ	HAEGEL	nature's natural disruptive force
ᚾ	NYD	need, compulsion, desire
ᛁ	IS	ice, stagnation, emotionless
ᛄ	GER	harvest, fruit, bloom, ripen
ᛇ	EOH	deflection, prevention
ᛈ	PEORTH	mystery, chance
ᛉ	EOLH	protection to grow, refuge
ᛋ	SIGIL	light, wholeness, discovery
ᛏ	TIR	courage, bravery
ᛒ	BEORC	rebirth, beauty, freshness, fertility
ᛖ	EH	speed
ᛗ	MAN	soul
ᛚ	LAGU	water, tide, cleansing
ᛝ	ING	love, peace, unity
ᛟ	ODAL	hearth, home
ᛞ	DAEG	day, breakthrough, dawning

Simple Three Rune Cast

Relax and think about what wisdom you may need or maybe choose a question for which you require insight.

Holding your runes in their bag, ask for their wisdom to be shown to you.

Lay out your cloth and choose the first rune from your bag.

RUNE 1 This rune is to give wisdom and to throw light upon your situation, or your question.

Choose a second rune from your bag.

RUNE 2 This rune shows you what is in front of you, possibly your challenge, or what you may need to face up to.

Choose a third rune from your bag.

RUNE 3 This rune is showing you what you may need to do now or in your near future.

When reading this rune cast it is important to allow your conscious and unconscious mind to help you understand. Reading runes can take practise so if at first it doesn't make sense to you, write the symbols down, date them, and if it feels good, draw it too. You can then revisit this reading in the future. The runes are ancient and will be with us forever, there is no rush.

I always thank the runes for their help.

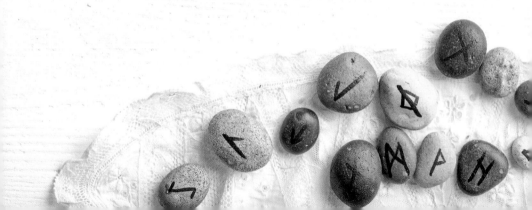

Black Sigil

Do you have an intention that needs to be held strongly? Do you need to feel strong? Perhaps you have been hunching your shoulders a little or hiding away. Maybe now is the time to push your shoulders back. You might not feel ready yet. But it will come. Black may well be the colour to support you. Remember, forming your intention with clarity will keep your desires crystal clear and make the spell stronger.

Breathe.

Decide on your intention or wish... for example, **I STAND TALL**.

Write your intention down on paper.

Remove the vowels and any repeated letters.

I̶ STA̶ND T̶A̶L̶L̶

Look at the letters you are left with and create your sigil.

S T N D L

Using a fresh black candle, take a pin and scratch your sigil onto your candle, maybe 2.5cm/1in below the wick.

To increase the power of your spell, place the candle on your altar.

Sprinkle a pinch of salt around your candle.

Breathe.

Light your candle.

As you watch it burn, stand straight and focus on your strength and intention.

When you feel ready, snuff out your candle.

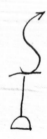

As with all magic, take a moment to breathe, make a note of your sigil and also note how you felt when you activated it. Resilient? Powerful? In control? Keep a record so you can see how long it takes for your intentions to materialize.

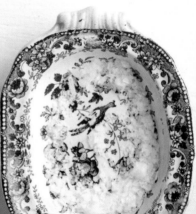

Grey Sigil

Grey, a traditionally calming colour, can help you seek answers and insight. Is there something a grey sigil could help you with? What could this mean for you?

Breathe.

Decide on your intention or wish, for example...
I LISTEN

Write your intention down on paper.

Remove the vowels and any repeated letters.
~~I LISTEN~~

Look at the letters you are left with and create your sigil.
L S T N

Take a beautiful, perfect grey pebble, the kind that fits well into the palm of your hand and feels lovely and smooth to the touch.

Breathe.

With chalk or chalk paint, inscribe your sigil on the pebble.

Keep the pebble in your pocket, on your altar or leave upon a beach.

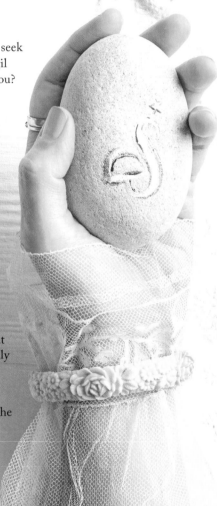

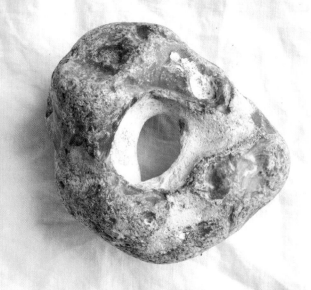

Hag Stone

A hag stone is any stone with a hole in the centre that has been formed naturally, usually by the flow of water. They are often found near beaches, brooks and rivers. Hag stones are also known as holey stones, witches' stones and fairy stones.

On the eve of a full moon, it is said that you can see the fairy realm through the hole.

Hag stones are reputed to have magical powers and are one of my favourite amulets. Tied to a bed post they are said to dispel bad dreams, protect from negative energy and keep the mischievous fey from disturbing our rest. Sailors and fishermen would seek them for safe passage and to this day, boats and trawlers are often seen with a stone charm tied to their hull.

Try threading a ribbon through one and tying it to your bedhead for sweet dreams.

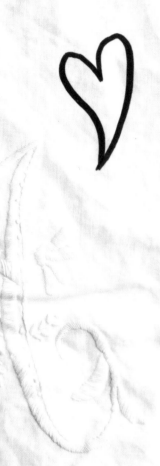
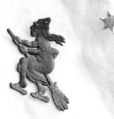

Witch's Heart

A witch's heart is quite distinctive, with a tail at the bottom that curves to the left or the right. These amulets have been worn since ancient times and are used to protect against bad spirits.

Traditionally worn on the left thigh during childbirth, they are said to aid safe delivery. They were gifted to nursing mothers as a charm to help their milk to flow and were also pinned to children's clothing to protect the infant from being 'stolen by the fairies'.

In the eighteenth century, witches' hearts were presented as a love token to imply that the giver had become bewitched by the recipient.

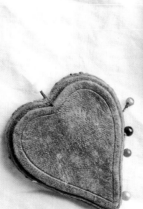
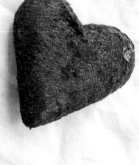

Pendulum

A pendulum is a wonderful and intuitive tool that can give a
YES or NO answer to a simple question. It's easy to make your
own. All you need is an object to weight the pendulum – such as
a ring, bead, charm or crystal – and something to tie it from. You
could use a thread, shoelace, chain, ribbon or length of string.

I always say thank you to the pendulum once it has given an
answer – I believe it's important to honour your tools and be
polite when performing magic.

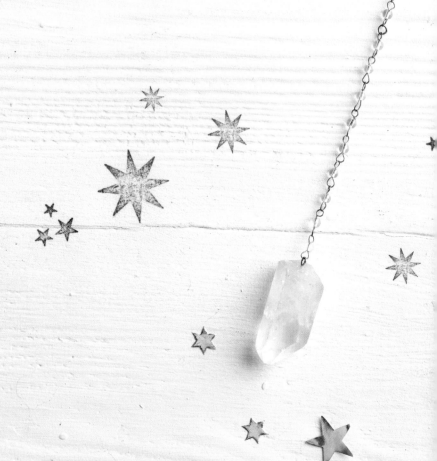

* Hold the thread or chain between your thumb and forefinger.

* Rest your elbow on a table.

* Make sure the thread is free to swing and the object is pointing down.

* Breathe.

* To ascertain the direction of YES and NO, focus, and ask your pendulum a question with an answer you already know to be *yes*.

* Your pendulum will begin to move in circles, or swing back and forth.

* Once you have noticed which way your pendulum is swinging for YES, stop the pendulum moving.

* Breathe.

* Ask the pendulum a question with an answer you already know to be *no*.

* Notice and note this, stop the pendulum moving again.

* When forming a question to ask, think carefully about what you really want to know.

* Ask your question and wait for an answer.

* Thank the pendulum for its wisdom.

You can also hold your pendulum over images and text to ask questions.

To clean your pendulum after use, simply 'wash' with incense smoke, pull the energy off the pendulum with your hand, making sure you throw this energy away from you. Recharging your pendulum with the moon can be done on any night, but for maximum effect, lay your pendulum on a windowsill or outside during the night of a full moon.

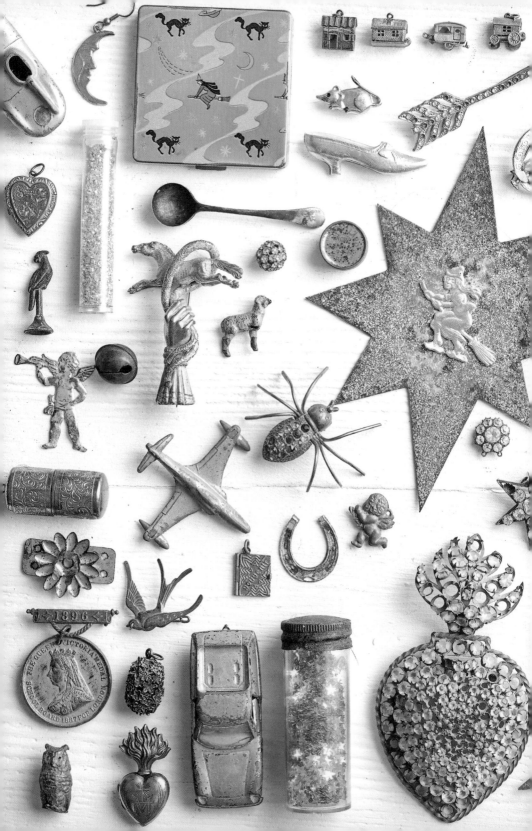

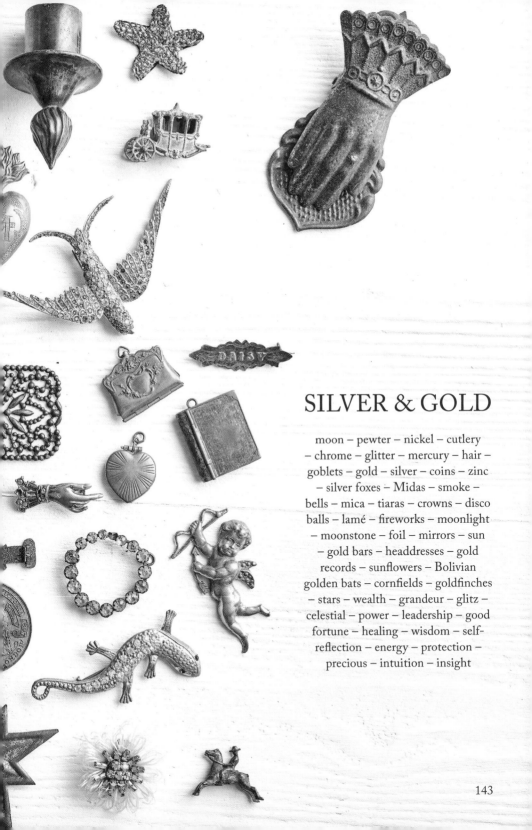

SILVER & GOLD

moon – pewter – nickel – cutlery
– chrome – glitter – mercury – hair –
goblets – gold – silver – coins – zinc
– silver foxes – Midas – smoke –
bells – mica – tiaras – crowns – disco
balls – lamé – fireworks – moonlight
– moonstone – foil – mirrors – sun
– gold bars – headdresses – gold
records – sunflowers – Bolivian
golden bats – cornfields – goldfinches
– stars – wealth – grandeur – glitz –
celestial – power – leadership – good
fortune – healing – wisdom – self-
reflection – energy – protection –
precious – intuition – insight

SILVER & GOLD

As far back as is recorded, gold and silver have been seen as precious, magical metals. While evoking images of wealth, grandeur and glitz, gold and silver are also revered as the celestial colours of the sun and moon.

In Japan, in a process called *kintsugi* or *kintsukuroi*, cracked pottery is repaired with a mixture containing real gold, transforming the object's cracks into a thing of beauty. The philosophy behind this beautiful act of repair is thought to celebrate the frailty of life and honour the ageing process. As with any act of healing, *kintsugi* is carried out with thought, care and honour.

Let the colour gold remind you that we shouldn't hide from the 'cracks' in our own lives. When we sometimes feel broken beyond repair it is important to acknowledge our wounds and to allow ourselves to heal with kindness. To have been broken is not a failure. To heal and repair ourselves takes courage and deserves a golden badge of honour.

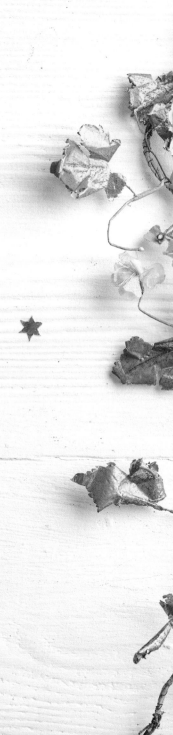

altar

flower: golden corn, silver fern
precious metals: silver, gold
element: water, fire

Silver is the colour and metal of the moon and many moon amulets are set into silver for this very reason. Silver talismans or charms are wonderful when you would like to ask the moon to help strengthen your intentions. It's also thought that turning silver coins over in your pocket beneath a full moon can increase your luck. (Remember, even if you cannot see the full moon because of clouds or rain, the moon's power is just as strong.)

Silver is associated with feminine intuition, healing and intense self-reflection and is often used when scrying (foretelling the future) as you gaze into water, smoke, a mirror or a crystal.

Gold and silver are traditionally fashioned into jewellery, charms and precious items.

Symbol Cloth

Our altar is our sacred space and it's lovely to make a symbol cloth to decorate it. These are particularly wonderful if you are travelling, as you can use this cloth to create a space for magic wherever you go or use it to transport your tools. Vintage handkerchiefs and napkins are great for this, especially damask linen.

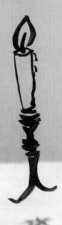

* cloth, such as a napkin or handkerchief
* star stamps
* silver and gold stamp ink
* needle and gold and silver thread

Stamp some star shapes across your cloth.

Allow to dry completely.

With your metallic threads you could add starbursts and delicate details such as magical symbols.

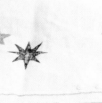

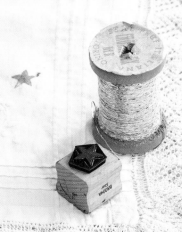

Charm Brooch

When sewing always stitch with purpose! I don't mean to just sew but to sew with magic – you are creating a talisman and it needs to be stitched with feeling. These make wonderful gifts for friends – you can add wishes just for them.

* fabric pieces and scissors
* pins, needles and safety pins

* threads (different colours)
* gold and silver beads and charms

From your cloth, measure and mark out two rectangles, each 3 x 5cm/1¼ x 2in, and cut them out. Pin and sew the rectangles together.

Choose a symbol – a star, a pentagram, a moon or sun, an anchor or four-leaf clover, an owl or a cat, initials or a word... This is a talisman and should provide the wearer with a feeling of protection.

Embroider the chosen symbol onto the front of your brooch.

Add some beads and a few charms (the charms should hang down from your brooch like they would on a medal).

Sew a safety pin to the back of your brooch along the top edge.

Add a few beads along the top, if you like.

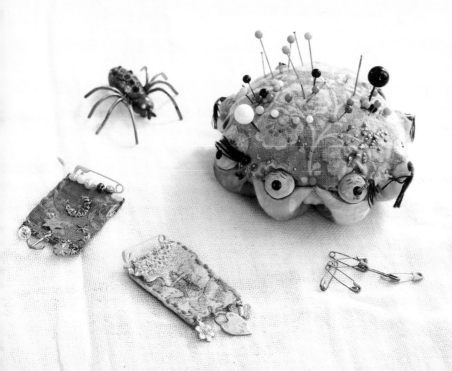

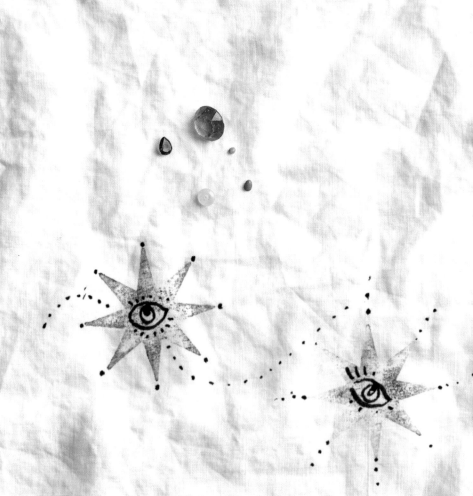

Secret Message Jewellery

Acrostic jewellery involves adding secret messages to a piece with gemstones. The art was thought to have been invented by Jean-Baptiste Mellerio, a jeweller at the French court of Versailles in the eighteenth century who attracted the patronage of Marie Antoinette with his cryptic, sentimental and romantic jewels. These delights found favour in the Georgian era but became more popular in Victorian times. Acrostic jewellery takes the first letter of each gem included in the piece to spell out a word and convey a secret message to the recipient. Popular words to include were…

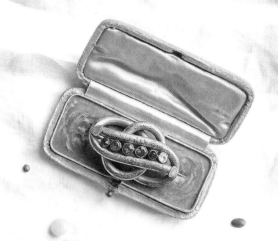

REGARD

R = ruby
E = emerald
G = garnet
A = amethyst
R = ruby
D = diamond

ADORE

A = amethyst
D = diamond
O = opal
R = ruby
E = emerald

AMOUR

A = amethyst
M = moonstone
O = opal
U = uraninite
R = ruby

Acrostic jewels were traditionally set in gold and feature precious and semi-precious jewels, although there were cheaper alternatives available made from brass or pinchbeck, set with glass stones.

DEAR

D = diamond
E = emerald
A = amethyst
R = ruby

Scry

*Scry - Foretell the future using a crystal ball or other
reflective object or surface.*
Oxford English Dictionary

To scry you will need a calm reflective surface to gaze into. This can be a mirror, a
crystal ball or even a natural pool, such as a rock pool, pond or slow-flowing stream.
(You can even try gazing into the flames of a gently burning fire, a calm sea, smoke
plumes – see page 36 – and dark shadows.)

For me, scrying is seeing or gazing into another world – the medium you are
looking into is a portal to that world. This can be very powerful. Sometimes shapes,
like faces or creatures, will appear in the corners of your vision for a fleeting
moment, and for me these shapes reveal treasured information, insight and answers
to my questions.

Scrying takes patience. It can take time to learn and practice will yield rewards
beyond your imagination. An ability to read symbols is also a great help. There are
many wonderful books that can help you with this.

* Take a moment to settle, maybe light a candle or some incense.
* When you feel ready and relaxed, gaze into your object or surface.
* Look beyond the reflection, as if your eyes are beginning to search
  for the unknown.
* Breathe.
* Look for unusual shapes or symbols or the shapes of the space
  between the light.
* If a symbol or face, creature or sign that you recognize begins to
  become clear, greet it and thank it for showing you its wisdom.
* Sometimes the symbols will be just beyond reach, but that's okay.
  Relax and keep looking.

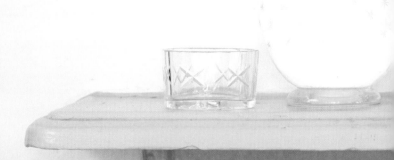

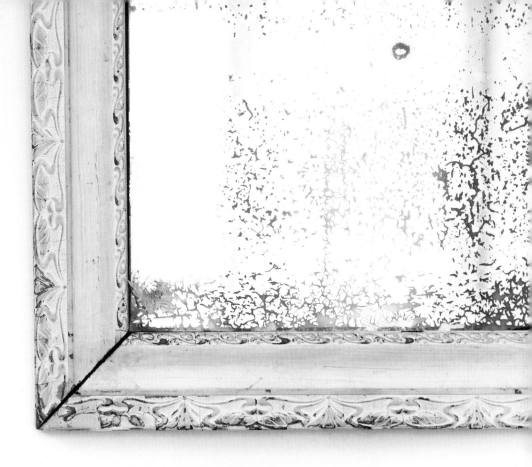

When you have finished, make a note
or draw what you saw. What does it
represent to you? Is there a message?

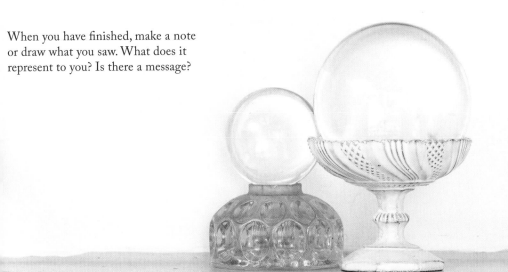

Welcome Little Stranger

The forthcoming birth of a new baby yields strong, earthy magic and even the most vehement non-believers will ponder on the unborn child's personality and future. Dreams, intuition and 'gut' feelings are often discussed at this expectant time.

We all have magic weaving through us.

In the eighteenth century, a baby was greeted with the phrase 'welcome little stranger'. Decorative pincushions made from silk, filled tightly with sand, with pins pushed in to form the words, were often gifted to expectant mothers as a token of love.

These cushions were placed in the unborn baby's crib or room until their birth, then the cushion would be hung on the front door of the house to serve as a joyous announcement of the arrival of the new little stranger.

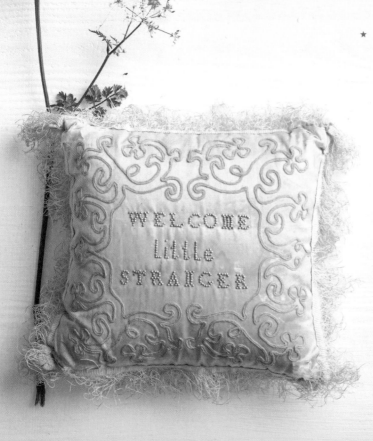

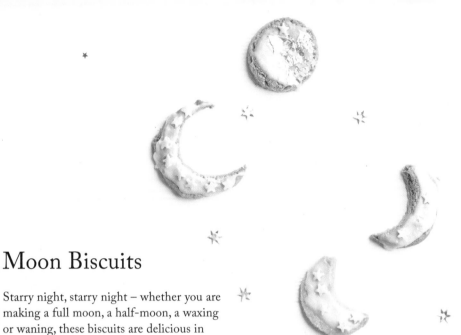

Moon Biscuits

Starry night, starry night – whether you are
making a full moon, a half-moon, a waxing
or waning, these biscuits are delicious in
their buttery, crumbly moreishness.

Makes about 20 biscuits

- ★ 100g/3½oz salted butter, plus extra for greasing
- ★ 50g/1¾oz/heaped ¼ cup caster sugar
- ★ 150g/5¼oz/scant 1¼ cups self-raising flour
- ★ 2 tbsp icing sugar
- ★ edible glitter, stars and foil

Preheat the oven to 160°C/140°C fan/315°F/gas mark 2–3.

Grease a baking tray with butter.

Beat the butter a little to soften it.

Add the sugar and flour and mix to form a smooth dough with your hands.

Divide the dough evenly into 14 pieces and form each one into a small ball.

Divide some of the balls in two, then flatten the dough with your palm and use
a knife to create waxing and waning crescent moons.

Flatten the other balls with your palm to create full moons.

Bake for 15–20 minutes until golden brown. Transfer to a wire rack to cool.

To make the icing, mix together the icing sugar with 1 tsp water.

Once cool, ice the biscuits and sprinkle with decorations.

Gold Sigil

Gold can be a powerful aid while creating a sigil. Invigorating and protective, gold is the perfect colour to use when focusing on moving forward, a journey, or if you feel stuck.

Breathe.

Decide on your intention or wish, for example...

I CAN

Remove the vowels and any repeated letters...

I̶ CA̶N

Look at the letters you are left with...

C N

Draw your sigil – remember you can add your own flourishes.

Try drawing the sigil onto the palm of your left hand in gold pen – the left palm often indicates your inner self.

Hold a golden object or symbol, such as a celestial star, in your hand as you focus on your intention.

Gold Candle

A gold candle represents the sun, strength, willpower and optimism. A protective colour for healing and blessings. A golden candle can be used in rituals requiring openness with the universe.

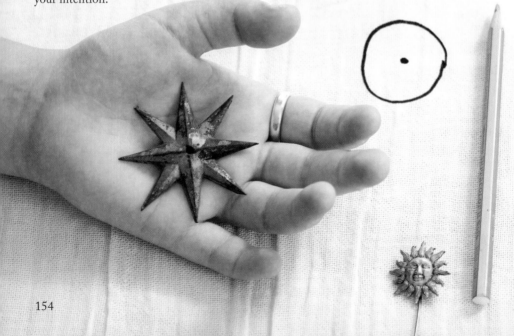

Silver Sigil

Let's add a little drama and try activating this sigil on the night of a full moon. This will still be productive on a cloudy night. Burn some incense in a fireproof bowl, outside or on a ledge beneath an open window, as you decide on your intention.

Take a moment

Breathe.

Decide on your intention or wish, for example...

I KNOW MY PATH

Write your intention down on paper.

Remove the vowels and any repeated letters...

I̶ KN̶O̶W MY PATH

Look at the letters you are left with...

K N W M Y P T H

Draw your sigil on a piece of paper in silver ink.

Burn your sigil carefully in your bowl – ask the moon for help and wisdom and it will guide you on your way.

Plant the ashes into the earth.

Silver Candle

A silver candle is often burned to represent the moon. Silver is linked with wish magic, communication with those that have passed and insight. The colour is said to represent the perfect balance between life and death.

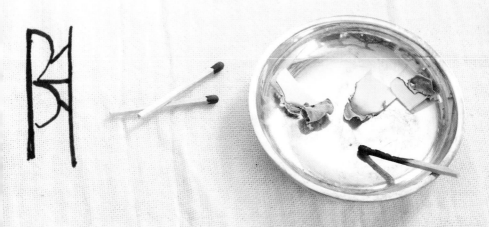

Diary Pages

Use these pages to record your sigils, dreams and insights.

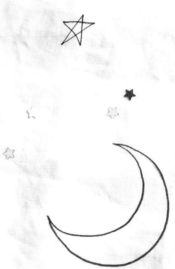

Resources

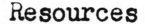

Although I am not part of a coven or group, I do reach out to witches, spirit guides and other experts – I am always learning and hope I always will. There are so many forms of magic and all of these can be explored.

To learn more

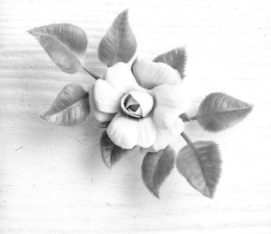

When travelling to meet your spirit animal, it is imperative to work with a qualified practitioner. I recommend Arya Ingvorsen.
www.amethysttiger.com

For online courses, learning, lectures and supplies I recommend Treadwell's Bookshop.
www.treadwells-london.com

For more information about British magical practice, I recommend The Museum of Witchcraft and Magic in Cornwall – it's an outstanding gem.
www.museumofwitchcraftandmagic.co.uk

For rainbow spell candles, I recommend Arcanus.
www.arcanus.co.uk

Natural Treasures

The natural world needs to be respected and protected. Treasures from the earth, from crystals and gems to flowers and feathers, are not an infinite resource. When decorating an altar with natural objects it is vital that we follow the less-is-more approach and prize quality over quantity, so curate a small collection that has special meaning for you. Always obtain your objects from sustainable, ethical sources, and repurpose existing objects whenever you can. Forage thoughtfully and be sure that the removal of the item you'd like to take will not harm the other species that live in that environment. For example, as tempting as it might be, never remove shells from the beach – they play an essential role in marine ecosystems.

Special thanks to...

Clare Conville, my literary agent and friend.

Pavilion, my publishers, Polly Powell, Sophie Allen, Helen Lewis, Katie Hewett and Kei Ishimaru.

Laura Russell, my art director, who leads me from clutter and helps me make beautiful pages.

The magical Krissy Mallett, my dream editor.

Tony Briscoe for the most beautiful photographs throughout this book and to Sharon Aston, for the exquisite photograph of the Cornish sea on page 95.

Bridgette Jones @moetlala for the loan of the Little Stranger cushion, @designersguild for the lovely green candles, @arya_ingvorsen for my journey, @janecountryroses for dried flowers, @splatteredinky for the best ribbons, and @rae_ceramics for her beautiful moon palette.

Especially and always to my family: Steve, my love, and my beautiful daughters, Daisy and Ruby.

SAM McKECHNIE

Sam McKechnie is an artist and doll maker. Her work is inextricably linked with fairy tales, magic and charms and has featured in many books and magazines across the globe. Sam created The Magpie & the Wardrobe atelier in 2002 as an extension of her art work. Through Magpie, she creates charm jewellery, fashion accessories and dolls, which are sold all over the world.

Sam can be reached via her Instagram pages @themagpieandthewardrobe.com or @sam_mckechnie_art

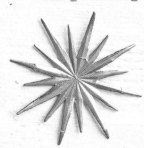

First published in the United Kingdom in 2022 by
Pavilion
43 Great Ormond Street
London
WC1N 3HZ

An imprint of Pavilion Books Company Ltd
Copyright © Pavilion Books Company Ltd
Text copyright © Sam McKechnie

ISBN: 978-1-911682-10-3

A CIP catalogue record for this book is available
from the British Library.

10 9 8 7 6 5 4 3 2 1

Reproduction by Rival Colour Ltd., UK
Printed and bound by Toppan Leefung
    Printing Ltd., China
Photographer: Tony Briscoe
Design Manager: Laura Russell
Commissioning Editor: Sophie Allen
Copy Editor: Krissy Mallett

www.pavilionbooks.com

FSC
www.fsc.org
MIX
Paper from
responsible sources
FSC® C104723

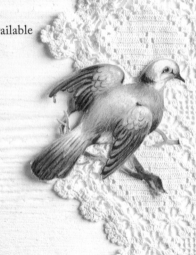

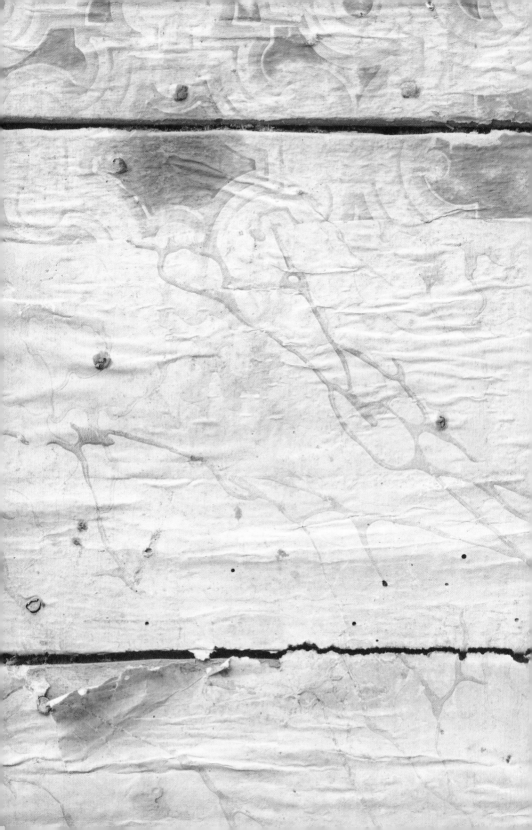